Mustapha SELLAMI
Samira ABDI

Nasosinusal polyposis and quality of life

Mustapha SELLAMI
Samira ABDI

Nasosinusal polyposis and quality of life

ScienciaScripts

Imprint

Cover image: www.ingimage.com

This book is a translation from the original published under ISBN 978-620-6-71645-7.

Publisher:
Sciencia Scripts
is a trademark of
Dodo Books Indian Ocean Ltd. and OmniScriptum S.R.L publishing group

120 High Road, East Finchley, London, N2 9ED, United Kingdom
Str. Armeneasca 28/1, office 1, Chisinau MD-2012, Republic of Moldova, Europe
Printed at: see last page
ISBN: 978-620-7-94386-9

Introduction

Chronic rhinosinusitis (CRS) is one of the most common pathologies in the world, affecting around 14% of people in the USA. [1]. It is defined by chronic inflammation of the nasosinus cavities lasting more than 12 weeks [2]. It may be with or without polyps.

Nasosinus polyposis (NSP) is a chronic rhinosinusitis characterized by multifocal, bilateral edematous degeneration of the mucosa of the lateral masses of the ethmoid, manifested clinically by the development of polyps in the nasal cavity. [3,4]

These polyps are the result of chronic inflammation of the nasosinus mucosa, with eosinophilic infiltration characteristic of the disease. [3]

PNS may be primary or secondary, isolated or associated with other pathologies such as asthma, intolerance to aspirin and NSAIDs, or Fernand Widal disease, which is known for its resistance to all therapies.

The prevalence of SNP is estimated at 4% in the general population, and is considered a pathology of the young adult. [5]

Its pathophysiology remains poorly elucidated, and several studies and theories have tried and are still trying to explain it. This obscure pathophysiology makes the aims of treatment not to cure this pathology, but rather to improve patients' functional symptomatology.

The recognized treatment for SNP is primarily medical, based on topical corticosteroids, interspersed with short courses of systemic corticosteroids.

Surgical treatment remains the last resort, after failure of medical therapy or contraindications to its use. Several surgical techniques have been used over the years to treat a condition that is known to be resistant to treatment and to recur despite optimal medical and surgical treatment. [[2,66-8]

References :

[1] M. S. Benninger *et al*, "Adult chronic rhinosinusitis: definitions, diagnosis, epidemiology, and pathophysiology," *Otolaryngol.--Head Neck Surg. Off. J. Am. Acad. Otolaryngol.-Head Neck Surg.* vol. 129, n° 3 Suppl, p. S1-32, Sept. 2003, doi: 10.1016/s0194-5998(03)01397-4.

[2] " European Position Paper on Rhinosinusitis and Nasal Polyps 2012. - PubMed - NCBI." https://www.ncbi.nlm.nih.gov/pubmed/22764607 (accessed May 16, 2019).

[3] P. Bonfils and Q. Lisan, "Apport de la chirurgie dans le traitement de la polypose nasosinusienne", *Bull. Académie Natl. Médecine*, vol. 203, n° 1-2, pp. 44-51, March 2019, doi: 10.1016/j.banm.2019.03.004.

[4] P. L. Larsen and M. Tos, "Origin of nasal polyps", *The Laryngoscope*, vol. 101, n° 3, pp. 305-312, March 1991, doi: 10.1288/00005537-199103000-00015.

[5] " Prevalence of asthma, aspirin intolerance, nasal polyposis and chronic obstructive pulmonary disease in a population-based study. - PubMed - NCBI." https://www.ncbi.nlm.nih.gov/pubmed/10480701 (accessed Nov. 09, 2019).

[6] D. W. Kennedy, S. J. Zinreich, A. E. Rosenbaum, and M. E. Johns, "Functional endoscopic sinus surgery. Theory and diagnostic evaluation," *Arch. Otolaryngol. Chic. Ill 1960*, vol. 111, n° 9, pp. 576-582, Sept. 1985, doi: 10.1001/archotol.1985.00800110054002.

[7] R. E. Gliklich and R. Metson, "Effect of sinus surgery on quality of life," *Otolaryngol.--Head Neck Surg. Off. J. Am. Acad. Otolaryngol.-Head Neck Surg.* vol. 117, n° 1, p. 12-17, July 1997, doi: 10.1016/s0194-5998(97)70199-2.

[8] J. R. Buckland, S. Thomas, and P. G. Harries, "Can the Sino-nasal Outcome Test (SNOT-22) be used as a reliable outcome measure for successful septal surgery?", *Clin. Otolaryngol. Allied Sci.* vol. 28, n° 1, p. 43-47, Feb. 2003, doi: 10.1046/j.1365-2273.2003.00663.x.

Chapitre 1 : History [9[9-11]

1.1 Development of rhinology through time :

The first publications on nasal polyps were found in Egyptian literature around 2000 BC.

By 1500 BC, the ancient Egyptians were already known for their familiarity and dexterity with the nasal cavity, as they regularly removed cranial contents through the nose to avoid facial disfigurement during the corpse mummification process.

Rhinological surgical procedures dating back to 700 BC are described in ancient Hindu and Egyptian medical publications. One of the great Hindu surgeons, Susruta, who practiced during the fifth century, was the founder of modern rhinoplasty and nasal reconstruction flaps.

Around the fifth century BC, although Susruta undertook advanced nasal surgery, Hippocrates (460-370 BC) was best known as the father of rhinology and medicine, due to his influence at a time when Greek civilization had reached its peak. In addition to establishing the "Hippocratic Oath", Hippocrates also observed and documented conditions related to otolaryngology, such as coryza, pharyngitis, intubation, uvulotomy, tonsillectomy, nasal fractures, epistaxis, sinusitis and nasal polyps.

Hippocrates called nasal growths "polyps" because of their resemblance to the marine polyp. This name has persisted to the present day. Hippocrates and other renowned physicians, including Claudius Galen, Paulus Aegineta and Fabricius Hildanus, were known in their day to have treated patients suffering from nasal polyps.

1.2 Development of etiopathogenesis :

Ideas on the pathophysiology of nasal polyps have also evolved.

Initially, polyps were thought to be due to a condition of thickened or viscous bodily secretions.

In the early centuries AD, Celsus and others noted that nasal polyps were influenced by wet weather and warm seasons.

The theory that these nasal tumors were a manifestation of systemic disease prevailed until the early 17th century, when it was assumed that local trauma contributed to their formation.

Boerhaave, in 1744, was among the first to assume that these outgrowths resulted from elongation of the linings of the membranes covering the sinuses.

Around the same time, Manne and Heister suggested that polyps arose as a result of obstruction of the mucous gland ducts.

The 19th century was also littered with controversy over the etiology of nasal polyps. Virchow and his pupils thought that these masses were primary tumors comprising myxomas and fibromas. Eggston and Wolff regarded them as passive mucosal edema, while others believed in an infectious etiology, with sinusitis or osteitis.

In 1843, Frerichs and Billroth surmised that polyps are really an enlargement of the normal nasal mucosa, as the epithelium covering the polyp was similar to the original sinus mucosa.

Systematic investigation of etiological associations began in the early 20th century. In 1933, Kern and Shenck proposed a relationship between allergy and nasal polyps, which was later invalidated.

Eggston, in his concept of polyp etiology, believed that polyps arose as a result of vascular changes in the nasal mucosa, induced by episodes of sinusitis. This would cause periphlebitis and obstructions in the interstitial tissue channels, preventing the return of extracellular fluid, leading to passive congestion and edema.

In the 1940s, advances in immunohistochemistry and immunobiology led to the first description of the predominance of eosinophils and lymphocytes in polyps.

Anderson and Bing showed that polyp stroma is a protein exudate, while Weisskopf and Burn considered it to contain mucopolysaccharides.

Berdal, thought that the extensive edema in polyps was due to allergic inflammation. However, Tandon and his team observed no difference in the histological appearance of allergic and infectious polyps.

Numerous other theories on the etiology of nasal polyps are under investigation today: bacterial infections, inflammation of the mucosa by bacterial superantigens, fungal inflammation, genetic factors (cystic fibrosis, primary ciliary dyskinesia) and aspirin hypersensitivity.

1.3 Diagnostic development :

Contrary to popular belief, the clinical description of nasal polyps was not limited to formations that protruded through the nostrils or formations that caused nasal deformities, but more than that.

In Egyptian literature, Samuel noted that a polyp manifests itself as a bad-smelling nose.

Hippocrates described polyps as pockets of mucus that caused nasal obstruction and disturbed the sense of smell.

Celsus attached polyps to the nipples of a woman's breast and wrote in his case reports that large polyps hung in the pharynx and on cold, wet days would strangle a man; describing large polyps that obstructed the choanae and oropharynx.

The development of the nasal speculum has considerably improved the examination of nasal cavities. While cauterizing patients for epistaxis, Hippocrates used a tubular speculum.

A similar prototype tubular speculum was also used by Hindu Ayurvedic (500) and Haly Abbas (940-980), a leading figure in Islamic medicine. These early speculums were modifications of instruments used in gynecology and rectal examinations. Fabricius Hildanus (1560-1634) made an auditory speculum that closely resembles the nasal speculum of modern times. Peret and Kramer improved the form of these instruments in the 18th century.

Sir Morell Mackenzie wrote that Levert, a French obstetrician, used a polished metal speculum that reflected sunlight to see polyps and tumors in the ears, throat and nostrils.

Until the 16th century, candlelight was mainly used to examine the nasal cavity. (**Figure 1**)

In the 1570s, Aranzii used a glass vial filled with water and candles to intensify the light directed into the patient's nose.

In 1829, a young physician named Benjamin Guy Babington presented a series of portable, angled mirrors to the Hunterian Medical Society and demonstrated the ability to reflect sunlight back into the pharynx. He also used a tongue retractor to obtain an unobstructed view. Although Babington decided before he could publish the success of his instruments in visualizing laryngeal structures, other authors mentioned his instruments and techniques.

Alfred Kirstein (1863-1922) is credited with introducing artificial light into the field. The instrument consisted of a flat spatula illuminated by a hand lamp.

Subsequently, Kirstein developed the first portable light, which bears a remarkable resemblance to those used today (**Figure 1**). Perhaps the biggest step was the advent of flexible optical fibers and rigid endoscopes in the late 1900s, which revolutionized the examination of the upper aerodigestive tract in otolaryngology.

The development of X-ray techniques in the 19th century also influenced the algorithm for diagnosing polyps.

Tomography, developed by Hounsfield in 1970, has surpassed conventional X-rays in providing superior imaging of the nasosinus cavities.

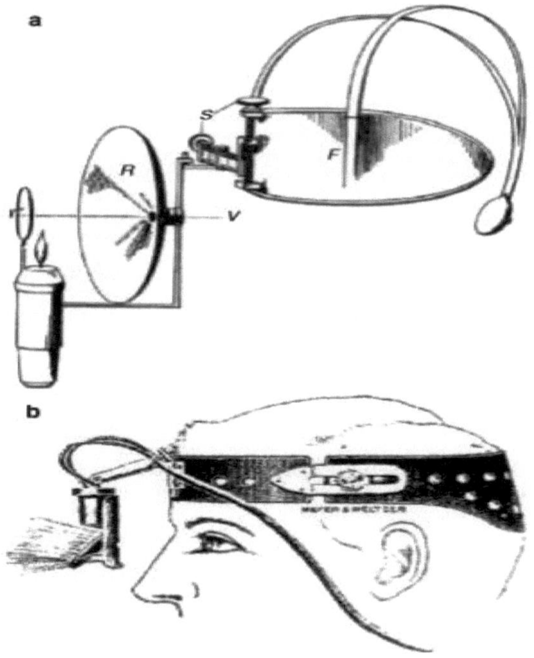

Figure 1 *Headlamps. (a). Adapted from Bailey and Weir, (b). Adapted from Kirstein.* [10] [12]

1.4 Treatment development :

The recurrent nature of nasal polyps has been known since the time of Hippocrates. Who wrote of patients requiring multiple treatments, and recognized that even after directed excision, additional therapy was required to prevent recurrence of these polyps. So, throughout history and right up to the present day, polyps have been treated both medically and surgically.

Hippocrates used nasal compresses and swabs coated with honey and copper salts to reduce the recurrence of polyps.

A Roman physician, Claudius Galen, treated polyps by applying fat, based on goose or calf fat and irritant medicines such as turpentine.

Antihistamines have been used as primary and post-surgical treatment for polyps.

The current mainstay of medical treatment is corticosteroids. The discovery of steroids marked a new era in the treatment of polyps.

Van Camp, was one of the first to describe the use of preoperative oral corticosteroid techniques to shrink polypoid tissue and facilitate its removal.

Intranasal steroids are widely used in the treatment of nasosinusal polyposis, and have been shown to reduce polyp size, delay recurrence and reduce the need for repeat surgery.

The history of surgical treatment of polyps is the most intriguing. In his treatises, Hippocrates describes several methods he used to remove polyps (**Figure 2**).

One of the methods employed was to use a sponge to bring the polyps back to its passage through the nasal cavity, a method used until the 1880s. He also used a hot iron passed through the nostrils to cauterize the polyps.

Aulus Cornelius Celsus, a renowned Roman physician also known as the Roman Hippocrates, frequently treated polyps with caustic agents, but also used a pointed spatula-like instrument to separate the polyp from the bone and pull it out of the nose with a hook-shaped instrument. The knotted chain method was used in the 6th and 7th centuries by Paulus Aegineta.

Before the Renaissance (1000-1200), Rolando, a famous Italian physician, also used knotted chain and spatula methods to remove polyps.

There was little change in surgical methods until 1600 and 1700, when knot clamps and forceps were developed (**Figure 3**).

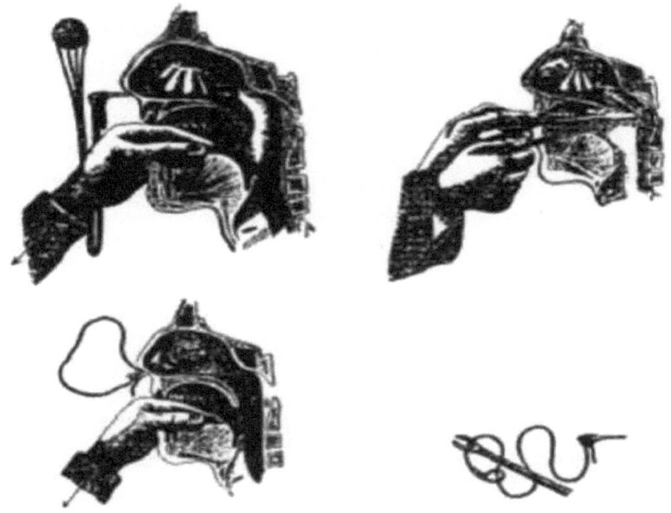

Figure 2*Hippocrates' method of polyp resection, after Stevenson and Guthrie.* [13] [10]

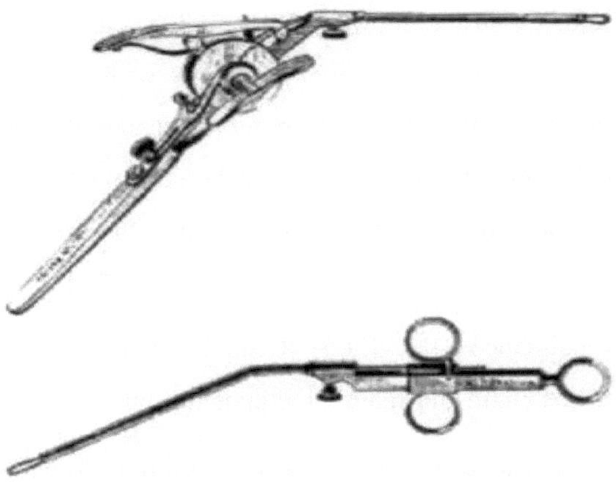

Figure 3*Node clamps*. [10]

Benjamin Bell, an eminent 18th-century Scottish surgeon, published a range of knot clamps and forceps for polyp removal in his System of Surgery (1791).

Throughout the 18th and 19th centuries, advances in the treatment of primary and recurrent nasosinus polyposis continued unabated. Until the use of endoscopy became popular, several endonasal procedures were used, such as the radical Caldwell-Luc antrostomy, endonasal ethmoidectomy and external fronto-ethmoidectomy.

Even with such extensive interventions and medical treatments, polyp recurrence remained a problem. This has led to significant changes in nasosinus surgery, with the development of endoscopic nasosinus surgery.

In 1901, Hirschman was the first to apply endoscopy to nasosinus disease.

In 1950, Storz introduced the first fiber-optic endoscope similar to those used today.

Despite technological advances, it wasn't until the 1960s that the endoscope gained in popularity for the diagnosis and surgical treatment of nasosinus diseases.

This new interest was due in part to the growing popularity of minimally invasive procedures in all surgical specialties, and in part to the work of Walter Messerklinger in Graz, Austria.

His work involved the anatomical and physiological study of the nose and paranasal sinuses with their mucosal covering.

More importantly, he noted the patterns of mucus clearance from different areas of the nose and sinuses, through various ostia and into the infundibulum, and that disruption of muco-ciliary transport or obstruction of normal outflow leads to the development of disease.

Thanks to Messerklinger's discoveries, Functional Endoscopic Sinus Surgery (FESS) was introduced in Germany in the late 1960s. And in 1985 in the USA, by David Kennedy.

The CO2 laser, already in use but of no interest, the YAG, Holmium and Diode laser, and KTP can sometimes stabilize the evolution without having to resort to surgery, particularly for recurrences.

Ultimately, nasal polyps have been around for a long time. Although many theories about their cause have evolved over the years, there is still much controversy and uncertainty about their etiology. Diagnosis and treatment strategies have undergone remarkable evolution. Nevertheless, to this day, the quest to cure nasal polyps remains an important objective, and new therapies will emerge to try and avoid the need for surgery in the management of these nasal polyps.

References :

[9] Peynegre, Freche, Fontanel, *la polypose naso sinusienne*. Société Française d'Oto-rhino-laryngologie et de Chirurgie de la Face et du Cou, 2000.

[10] T. M. Önerci and B. J. Ferguson, eds, *Nasal Polyposis: Pathogenesis, Medical and Surgical Treatment*. Berlin Heidelberg: Springer-Verlag, 2010.

[11] Mahassine EL HARRAS, "la polypose nasosinusienne: place de la chirurgie endonasale", Université CADI AYYAD, Marrakech, 2011.

[12] Bailey B, "What's all the fuss about? The laryngoscope pages cause an international incident", *Laryngoscope*, vol. 8, n° 106, pp. 939-943, 1996.

[13] Stevenson RS. and Guthrie D., "A history of otolaryngology", *Living Stone, Edinburgh*, pp. 70-71, 1949.

Chapitre 2 : Embryological background : [11, 14-17]

From the fourth week of embryonic development, nasal fossa development occurs in conjunction with the growth of the palate, facial skull and cerebral skull, more specifically the fronto-nasal apophysis. [18-20]

As the nasal cavity grows, three ectodermal elevations can be recognized on its lateral wall, giving rise to the turbinates and certain sinus cavities. [21-24]

The organogenesis of rhinosinus structures passes through three stages: mesenchymal, cartilaginous and bony. [25]

2.1 Mesenchymal stage :

At the end of the first month, the anterolateral part of the stomodeum shows an oval thickening, giving rise to two olfactory placodes. The latter two invaginate into the underlying mesoderm, giving rise to the olfactory gutters bounded by the internal and external nasal buds.

The nasal and maxillary buds join to form the primary palate, while the secondary palate results from the union of the maxillary buds and the palatal process. During the 6th week of embryonic life, this partitioning results in a primitive oral cavity and two nasal cavities. (**Figure 4**)

2.2 Cartilage stage :

Around the 9th week, cells from the neural crests progressively form condensation nuclei within the inner and outer nasal folds. Raised formations and recessed cavities are formed (**Figure 5**).

Laterally, the nasal capsule gives rise to beads, which are the future inferior, middle and superior turbinates, unciform processes and bullae. (**Figure 6**)

Unlike protrusions, invaginations are at the origin of the future anterior fronto-ethmoidal complex, maxillary sinus and posterior ethmoidal sinus.

The mucous membrane from the olfactory gutter penetrates the neurocranium, revealing the outline of the sphenoidal sinus.

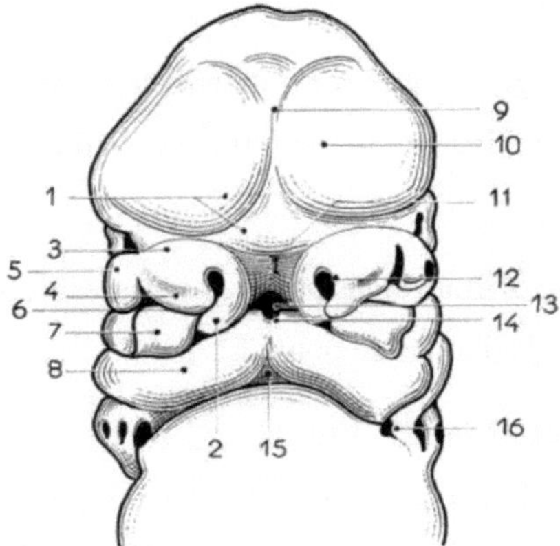

***Figure** 4Human embryo seen from the front.* [26]

1 and 3 Inner and outer frontal buds - 2 and 4 Inner and outer nasal buds - 5 Eye - 6 Tear duct - 7 and 8 Upper and lower maxillary buds - 9 Inter-hemispheric groove -10 Cerebral hemisphere - 11 Nasal cavity roof - 12 Nostril orifice - 13 Palatine gutter - 14 Primitive mouth - 15 Inter-maxillary groove - 16 2nd branchial arch (from Terracol).

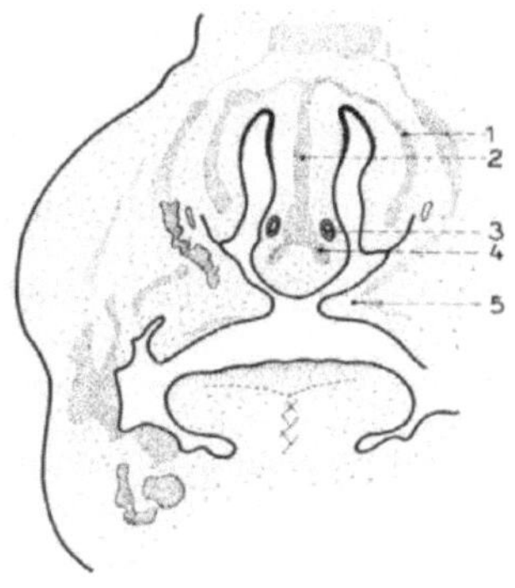

Figure 5*Frontal section of the cephalic region of a 9-week-old embryo.* [27]

1 Cartilaginous nasal capsule - 2 Nasal septum - 3 Jacobson's organ - 4 Vomeronasal cartilage - 5 Palatal bud (From Terracol)

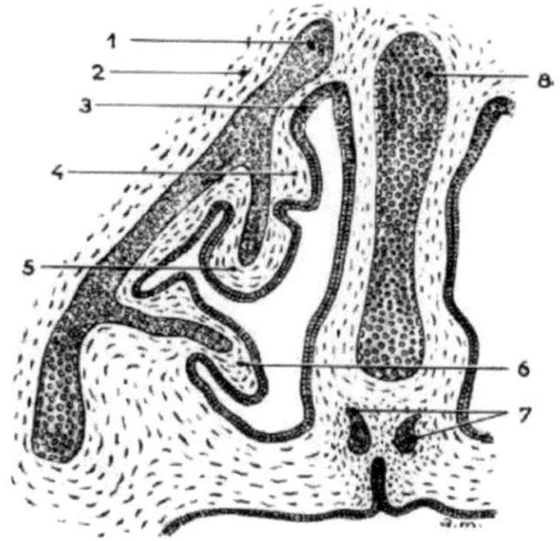

Figure 6*Horn formation.* [27]

1 Nasal capsule - 2 Mesenchyme - 3 Olfactory epithelium - 4, 5 and 6 Upper, middle and lower turbinates - 7 Para-septal cartilage - 8 Nasal septum.

2.3 Bone stage :

From the 4th month onwards, the cartilaginous structures ossify. The cells are divided into two groups: the anterior group in front of the dividing root, and the posterior group behind it.

The phenomenon of invagination and pneumatization leads to the formation of a true ethmoidal beehive (24-32 weeks).

By mid-gestation, the turbinate structures are individualized and the sphenoid is represented by a cartilaginous block with no pneumatization. **(Figure 7)**

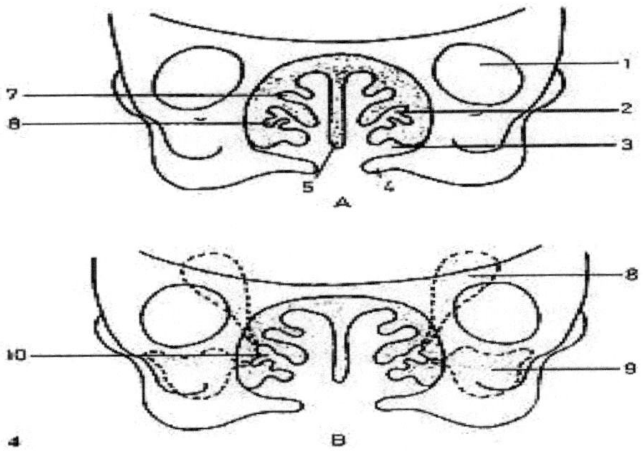

Figure *7Frontal sections of the embryonic nasal cavities.* [28]

A Paleo-sinus stage - B Neo-sinus stage.

1 Orbit - 2 Ethmoid-frontal recess - 3 Lower nasal meatus - 4 Palatine process - 5 Nasal septum - 6 Ethmoid-maxillary recess - 7 Upper nasal meatus - 8 Frontal sinus - 9 Maxillary sinus - 10 Middle nasal meatus.

2.4 Postnatal growth:

Classical embryology considers the formation of the ethmoid during the embryonic period. After birth, the already-ventilated ethmoidal cells would be responsible for the formation of the paranasal sinuses through colonization of the maxillary, sphenoidal and frontal bones.

The frontal sinus develops from the anterior ethmoid from the first year of life until adolescence.

The maxillary sinus is a shallow cavity that develops into a pyramid-shaped cavity around the age of 6-8.

The sphenoidal sinus begins to develop around the age of one, and continues into adolescence.

However, this concept of the ethmoidosinusal set does not explain certain anatomical data.

In the evo-devo concept, the paranasal sinuses (maxillary, sphenoidal and frontal) do not develop from the ethmoid. Their formation is the result of biological pneumatization mechanisms, as in the case of the mastoid cells of the human rock. It is a post-natal degeneration of the red marrow of the sphenoidal, maxillary and frontal bones, and its replacement by air cavities that become the maxillary, sphenoidal and frontal sinuses. [29-31]

2.4.1 Ethmoidal cells:

Around the 7th week of fetal life (1st trimester of pregnancy), which is the embryonic period of organogenesis, the ethmoid appears as the outline of a cartilaginous olfactory capsule surrounding the primary olfactory organ.

The primary olfactory organ appears in the embryo through invagination of the olfactory placodes towards the primary cerebral vesicle.

This cartilaginous olfactory capsule is phylogenetically derived from the prechordal cartilage of the first marine vertebrates (agnathans), for whom it already had the function of forming a protective skeleton around the olfactory mucosa.

In humans, the ethmoid is compartmentalized on either side of the median septum into an olfactory cleft, where the olfactory mucosa persists in the olfactory cleft beneath the cribriform lamina of the ethmoid, and an ethmoidal labyrinth, in which the olfactory mucosa has been replaced by vestigial mucosa.

2.4.2 Maxillary sinus :

This is the first to appear following an evagination of the lateral wall of the nasal cavities, below the middle turbinate and below the upper insertion of the lower turbinate (lower end of the uncibullar gutter; fontanel zone and location of a possible middle meatotomy).

This "mucus-filled cleft" increases in volume as it penetrates the body of the jawbone. The eruption of the first molar facilitates this amplification, which is completed after the eruption of the permanent dentition and the retraction of the facial skull.

It must be stressed that dysgenesis of the maxillary sinuses is possible, with the presence of gender differences (smaller volume in women than in men), and the possibility of acquiring a certain asymmetry in adulthood (the left always being more voluminous than the right).

2.4.3 The frontal sinus :

It is the result of pneumatization from the initial diverticulum, which originates in the anterior ethmoid. Its development begins in the sixth month of intrauterine life, but it does not invade the frontal bone until the first month after birth.

This evolution of the frontal sinuses can be hindered, giving rise to agenesis, which can be pure, by complete arrest of development, or trabecular or spongy, by incomplete arrest of development.

This cancellous agenesis is of a different etiology, as the "blowing" process has taken place but the frontal bone has not responded with a corresponding osteolytic process.

This notion is important, as frontal sinus agenesis is relatively frequent in unilateral forms, and their radiological interpretation is not unequivocal. [32]

2.4.4 The sphenoidal sinus :

The sphenoidal sinus is in place before birth (rostral center); by the fifth year, it invades the presphenoid, and by puberty, it has practically reached its final volume.

The formation of the sphenoidal sinus is intrinsically the result of a primary cavitation phenomenon in bone. These facts call into question Zukerkandl's century-old theory that ethmoidal cells have the power to expand and even colonize bone. Some authors have sought to demonstrate an "osteoclastic background" at the level of the "ethmoidal epithelial diverticula" to explain the hollowing of the facial bones, but the physiological inducing and regulating mechanisms of such behaviour of the ethmoidal mucosa are difficult to infer from its primitive nature.

References :

[11] Mahassine EL HARRAS, "la polypose nasosinusienne: place de la chirurgie endonasale", Université CADI AYYAD, Marrakech, 2011.

[14] F. Legent, L. Perlemuter, Cl. Vandenbrouck, *Cahiers d'anatomie ORL*, 4e ed., vol. 2. Masson, 1986.

[15] SOULTANA RABIE, "nasosinusal polyposis: experience of the ENT department at Moulay Ismail Hospital in Meknes (à propos de 60 cas)", Université Sidi Mohammed ben Abdellah, FES, 2015.

[16] M. ZAHIR ILIAS, " LA MEATOTOMIE MOYENNE DANS LE TRAITEMENT CHIRURGICAL DES SINUSITES MAXILLAIRES CHRONIQUES (à proposde55 cas) ", université Fès, maroc, 2018.

[17] Collectif, C. Freche, and J.-P. Fontanel, *L'obstruction nasale*. Paris: Arnette Blackwell, 1996.

[18] W. Larsen, P. R. Brauer, G. C. Schoenwolf, and P. Francis-West, *Human embryology*. De Boeck Superieur, 2017.

[19] G. Pradal and F. Resche, *Embryologie humaine élémentaire: L'individu de sa naissance à sa mise au monde*. Paris: Ellipses Marketing, 2005.

[20] T. W. Sadler, "Embryologie médicale (9e édition française - 13e édition américaine)". https://www.jle.com/fr/ouvrages/e-docs/embryologie_medicale_9e_edition_francaise_13e_edition_americaine__309597/ouvrage.phtml (accessed March 26, 2019).

[21] J. Foucrier, R. Franquinet, and M. Vervoort, *Atlas d'embryologie descriptive*, 3rd ed. Paris: Dunod, 2013.

[22] L. R. Cochard, *Netter's Atlas of human embryology*. De Boeck Superieur, 2015.

[23] J.-M. Retbi and T. W. Sadler, *Langmann's Atlas of Medical Embryology*, 1re ed. Rueil-Malmaison: Pradel, 2008.

[24] U. Drews, *Atlas de poche d'embryologie*. Paris: Flammarion Médecine-Sciences, 1994.

[25] E. Masson, "Embryology and congenital anomalies of the nose", *EM-Consulte*. https://www.em-consulte.com/article/64045/embryologie-et-anomalies-congenitales-du-nez (accessed March 28, 2019).

[26] J. Terracol and P. Ardouin, *Anatomie Des Fosses Nasales Et Des Cavités Annexes*, Librairie Maloine. 1965.

[27] Y. Guerrier and P. Rouvier, "Ostéologie Du Nez Et Des Sinus", *Encycl Méd Chir Oto-rhino-laryngologie*.

[28] J. M., C. Martin, and J. C. Balique, "De la pneumatisation cranio-faciale chez le foetus", *jornal Francais d'ORL*, vol. 1, n° 42, p. 11 6 20, 1993.

[29] R. Jankowski, *Du dysfonctionnement naso-sinusien chronique au dysfonctionnement ostio-meatal*. Paris: Société Française d'Oto-rhino-laryngologie et de Chrurgie de la Face et du Cou, 2006.

[30] R. Jankowski, *The Evo-Devo Origin of the Nose, Anterior Skull Base and Midface*. Paris: Springer-Verlag, 2013.

[31] R. Jankowski, C. Perrot, D. T. Nguyen, and C. Rumeau, "Structure of the lateral masses of the ethmoid by curved stacking of the endoturbinals", *Ann. Fr. Oto-Rhino-Laryngol. Pathol. Cervico-Faciale*, vol. 133, n° 5, pp. 293-298, Nov. 2016, doi: 10.1016/j.aforl.2016.02.010.

[32] S. Kuntzler, "At the frontiers of sinus development: from pneumatization arrest to pneumosinus dilatans", Oct. 2012, Accessed: Nov. 26, 2019. [Online]. Available from: https://hal.univ-lorraine.fr/hal-01734223.

Chapitre 3 : Anatomy of the nasosinus cavities: [11, 14-16]

3.1 Descriptive anatomy : [33-42]

3.1.1 Nasal cavities :

The nasal cavities or nasal fossae are two anfractuous cavities located in the middle of the upper facial mass, above the bony oral cavity, below the base of the skull, between the two orbital cavities. They are separated by a sagittal partition, the nasal septum, and protected at the front by the nasal pyramid. They open into the rhinopharynx at the back via the choanae, and at the front to the outside via the nostrils.

Each nasal cavity has four walls: lateral, medial or nasal septum, inferior or floor and superior or ceiling.

-The floor:

Forming a horizontal gutter with a smooth surface, its two anterior thirds are formed by the palatal process of the maxilla, while its posterior third is formed by the horizontal blade of the palate (**Figure 8**).

-The ceiling :

This wall can be broken down from front to back into three zones (**Figure 8**):

- A fronto-nasal zone formed by the posterior surface of the nasal bone, the frontal bone at the level of the spine and the medial part of the frontal sinus.
- An ethmoidal zone formed by the sieve plate of the ethmoid at the front and the ethmoidal process of the sphenoid at the back.
- A sphenoidal zone, where the sphenoidal sinus opens.

-Medial wall :

It consists of a skeleton comprising three osteo-cartilaginous parts (**Figure 8**):

- The perpendicular blade of the ethmoid, located in front of the upper part of the vomer, joins below and in front with the septal cartilage.
- The vomer, which takes up the posterior part of the nasal septum.
- The quadrangular or septal cartilage of the nose, in front.

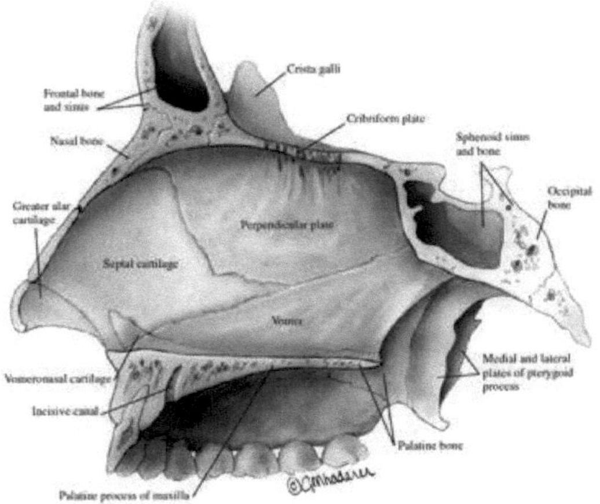

Figure 8*Skeleton of the septum (sagittal section).* [39]

C. septal cartilage - E. perpendicular blade of the ethmoid - V. vomer.

-Side panel :

It is formed by the assembly of bony pieces that form a wall tormented by significant reliefs and dehiscences, particularly in its central part. It has two levels:

An upper or ethmoidal stage separating the nasal fossa from the orbit

A lower or maxillary level, which separates the nasal fossa from the maxillary sinus at the front, and from the pterygo-maxillary fossa at the back.

This wall is divided into three regions in relation to the turbinates:

- A pre-turbinal region.

- A supraturbinal region.

- The turbinal region, the largest, represents three quarters of the lateral wall and includes the turbinates and meatus:

- **Cones:**

They are thin, obliquely-inward-slanting bony blades, rolled up on themselves in a laterally concave curve. (**Figure 9**)

Each cone contains :

-An enlarged anterior end or head of the horn.

-A fusiform body.

-A posterior end or tail of the horn, of variable shape.

Inconsistent rudimentary turbinates are added to the three constant turbinates: lower, middle and upper.

- **Meats:**

For each horn, there is a longitudinal gutter delimited by the corresponding part of the lateral wall called the meatus.

There are three main meats corresponding to the main turbinates:

-The inferior meatus, considered to be the lacrimal meatus.

-The middle meatus, a true crossroads of the anterior sinuses, where the maxillary sinus, frontal sinus and anterior ethmoidal cells open. Its middle segment features two reliefs, the unciform process and the bulla, two uncibullar and retrobullar gutters, and the cell orifices.

-The superior meatus is where the posterior ethmoidal cells open.

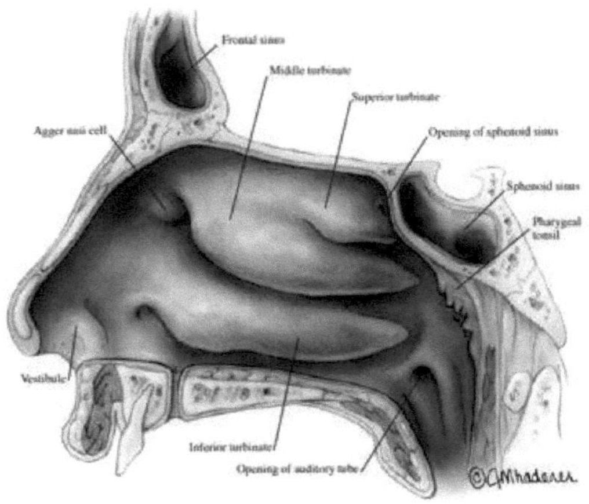

***Figure** 9Lateral wall of the left nasal cavity.* [39]

-Vascularization:

The mucosa of the nasal cavity is richly vascularized, with a blood system comprising intramucosal networks, arteries and veins, and a lymphatic system.

- **The blood system :**
  - **Intramucosal networks:** located in the chorion.

- The arterial network is made up of a deep network and a superficial network.

- The venous network, which is much more highly developed than the previous one, and is also made up of a superficial and a deep network.

- The capillary network, made up of a sub-epithelial network and a peri-glandular network.

The particularity of the respiratory mucosa lies in the presence of cavernous tissue, en bloc devices and arteriovenous anastomoses. Disruption of this vascularization is at the root of hypertrophic rhinitis.

- **Arterial irrigation:**

Assured by an arterial contingent from the internal and external carotids, with an anastomosis of these two systems at the level of the vascular spot. **(Figure 10)**

- **The internal carotid system :**

It vascularizes the nasal cavities via the anterior and posterior ethmoidal arteries, branches of the ophthalmic artery. These two arteries predominate in the vascularization of the upper and outer parts of the nasal cavity.

- **The external carotid system :**

The spheno-palatine artery, a branch of the maxillary artery, and the facial artery play the most important role.

The spheno-palatine artery, as it emerges from the spheno-palatine foramen, gives rise to two branches, one lateral or artery of the turbinates, the other medial or artery of the septum.

The facial artery gives rise to the superior labial artery, which, after anastomosis with its contralateral counterpart, gives rise to the superior coronary arch, then the artery of the nasal wing. This arcade gives rise to a branch destined for the septum or sub septum artery.

All these arteries anastomose with each other, providing sometimes formidable suppletions in the event of epistaxis. The most important of these anastomoses is the vascular spot, described at the end of the 19th century by Little and Kiesselbach. This is a zone of terminal branches of the anterior palatine, nasopalatine, anterior ethmoidal and subclavian arteries.

Another zone of anastomosis is Woodruff's zone, located on the underside of the lateral wall of the nasal cavity, behind the inferior turbinate. It is formed from the anastomosis of the spheno-palatine artery and the pharyngeal arteries. Its posterior position makes it a common source of severe non-traumatic bleeding. [43]

- **Venous drainage :**

Following three routes: anterior, into the angular vein; posterior, into the maxillary or pterygoid venous plexus; superior, into the ophthalmic vein.

- **The lymphatic system :**

Consists of superficial and deep intramucosal networks.

-Innervation: three types:

The innervation of general sensitivity is dependent on the V, via two trunks: the ophthalmic via the naso-ciliary nerve, and the maxillary via the pterygo-palatine nerves.

Vegetative innervation by the sympathetic and parasympathetic systems, via the pterygo-palatine ganglion.

Sensory innervation by the olfactory nerve.

3.1.2 Facial sinuses :

3.1.2.1 The ethmoidal sinus :

The ethmoidal labyrinth, or ethmoidal sinus, is a set of pneumatic cavities or cells hollowed out of the thickness of the lateral mass of the ethmoid, opening into the nasal cavities at the level of the middle and upper meatus.

According to Mouret's ethmoidal systematization, based on the anatomy of the turbinates and their extensions into the labyrinth, the partitioning root of the middle turbinate divides the labyrinth into two compartments:

anterior and posterior. (**Figure 11**)

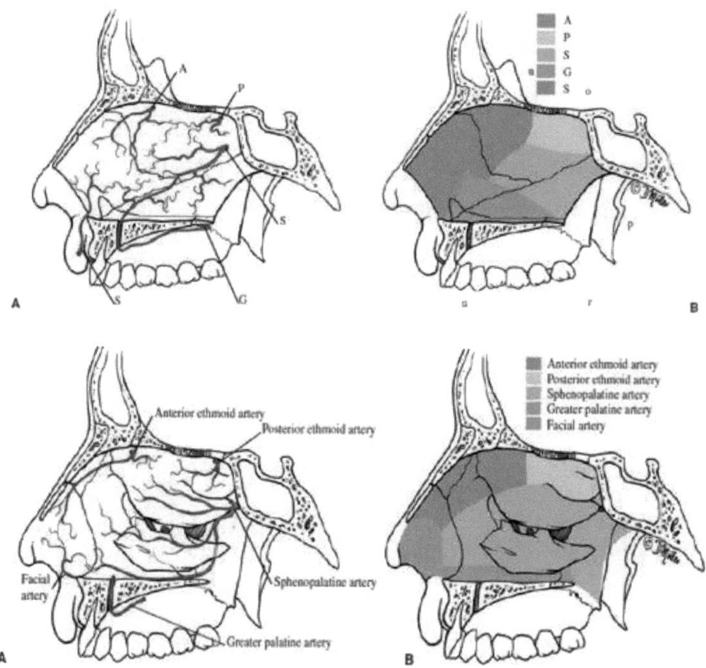

Figure 10*Vascularization of the nasal cavity. A. Vascular branches. B. Vascular territory.* [39]

1. Subclavian artery - 2. anterior ethmoidal artery - 3. cribriform lamina - 4. posterior ethmoidal arteries - 5. spheno-palatine artery - 6. spheno-palatine foramen - 7. posterolateral arteries - 8. internal maxillary artery.

- **Anterior ethmoid :**

Divided in turn by the partitioning roots of the unciform and bulla, resulting in three cellular systems:

-The bulla system contains one to three cells, including the ethmoido-maxillary cell, which opens into the retrobullary gutter.

-The unciform system contains several cells, including the almost constant agger nasi, which opens into the uncibullar gutter.

-The middle meatus system itself usually contains a single cell.

All the cells of the anterior ethmoid open into the middle meatus.

- **Posterior ethmoid :**

Comprised of three to five cells that open into the superior meatus, the septate root of the superior turbinate mimics the posterior ethmoid in two systems:

A main system draining into the upper meatus.

A fickle accessory system draining into the supreme meatus.

- **Reports :**

The ethmoidal labyrinth responds: (**Figure 12**)

Above, at the floor of the frontal sinus, and at the anterior level of the skull base,

Inward, to the upper half of the nasal cavity,

At the bottom, it overhangs the lower part of the middle meatus,

In front, it responds to the frontal process of the maxilla,

Externally, it connects with the lacrimal sac and orbital contents,

Posteriorly, the anterior surface of the sphenoid body.

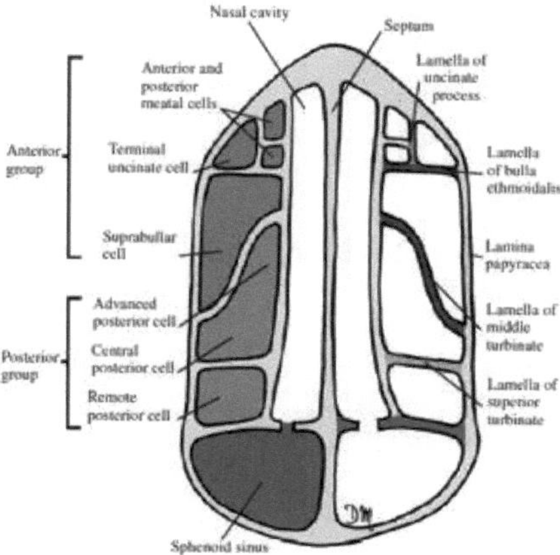

Figure 11*Systematization of the ethmoid according to Terrier*. [39]

- **Vascularization:**

It is supplied by the anterior and posterior ethmoidal arteries, branches of the internal carotid artery via the ophthalmic artery. They run beneath the ethmoid roof in bony canals that are sometimes dehiscent. (**Figure 13**)

Veins enter the cavernous sinus, facial vein and pterygoid plexus.

Lymphatics join the nasal and meningeal lymphatic system.

The trigeminal-sympathetic system of the nasal cavities and the anterior and posterior ethmoidal nerves innervate the ethmoid.

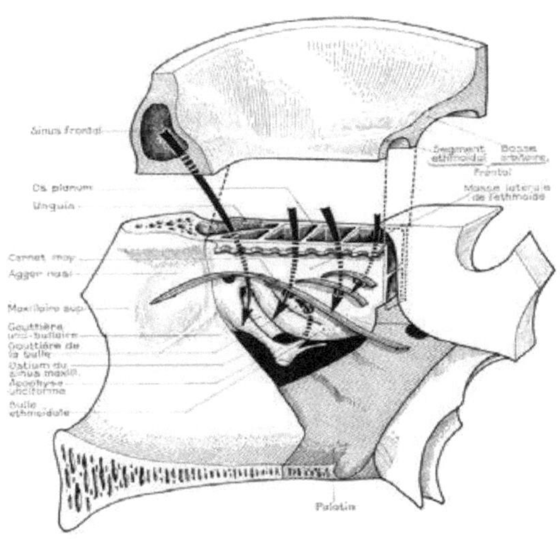

Figure 12*Internal, posterior and superior relationships of the right ethmoidal carter (after Perlemuter & Legent).* [14]

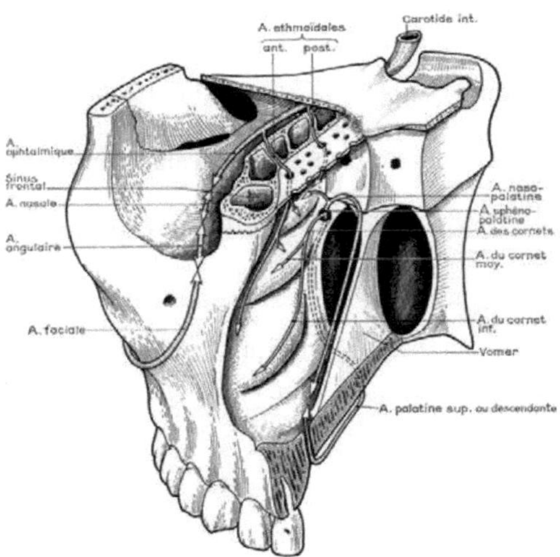

Figure 13*Right ethmoid anatomical relationship and vascularization (after Perlemuter & Legent).* [14]

3.1.2.2 The maxillary sinus :

This is a pneumatic cavity in the body of the maxilla. It is shaped like a triangular pyramid. (**Figure 14**)

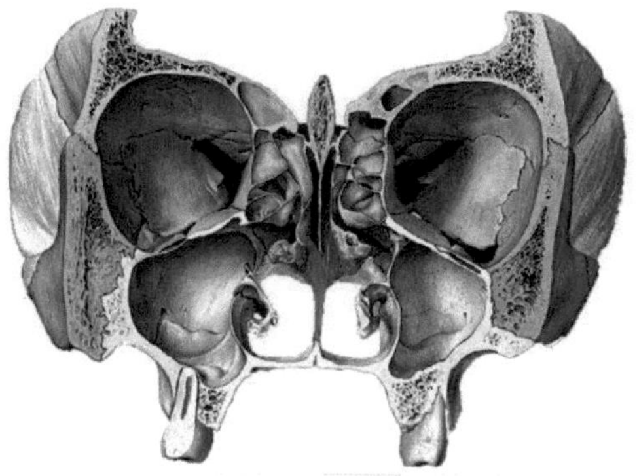

Figure 14*Frontal section through the maxillary sinuses.* [39]

It is distinguished by :

- Anterior or jugal wall:

This wall is surgically accessed from the outside, and is bounded at the top by the inferior orbital rim, medially by the anterior edge of the maxillary body, laterally by the buttress of the zygomatic bone, and inferiorly by the alveolar rim from the canine to the second premolar.

It features two important landmarks: The canine fossa and the infraorbital foramen. This wall is criss-crossed by nerve channels for the dental nerves and vascular channels. This wall is crossed by the upper vestibular cul de sac, giving two zones: lower or gingivobuccal, and upper or jugal.

- A posterior wall :

Answering the maxillary tuberosity separating the sinus from the pterygo-maxillary fossa, looking back and out, 2 mm thick, it is crossed by the superior and posterior dental nerve canal on the outside, and the accessory palatine and palatine canals on the inside.

-A top wall :

Triangular in shape with a posterior apex, particularly thin and fragile, this wall forms the floor of the orbit, divided in two by the gutter and the infraorbital canal, and is in contact with the orbital contents.

- A medial wall :

An endoscopic surgical wall, it corresponds to the inter-sinus-nasal septum, forming the lower half of the lateral wall of the nasal cavity, between the frontal process of the maxilla in front and the perpendicular blade of the palatine behind.

It is divided into two regions by the insertion of the inferior turbinate: anteroinferior, corresponding to the inferior meatus, and posterosuperior, corresponding to the middle meatus.

- A floor :

It corresponds to the depressed part of the channel-shaped sinus, slightly below the level of the floor of the nasal cavity. Dental sockets protrude into this area, mainly those of the first and second molars and second premolars. **(Figure 15)**

- Superior-medial angle:

The maxillary sinus ostium is located between the medial and superior walls, where the maxillary sinus meets the ethmoidal sinus at its inferolateral edge. The ostium is located where the anterior and middle thirds of the angle meet.

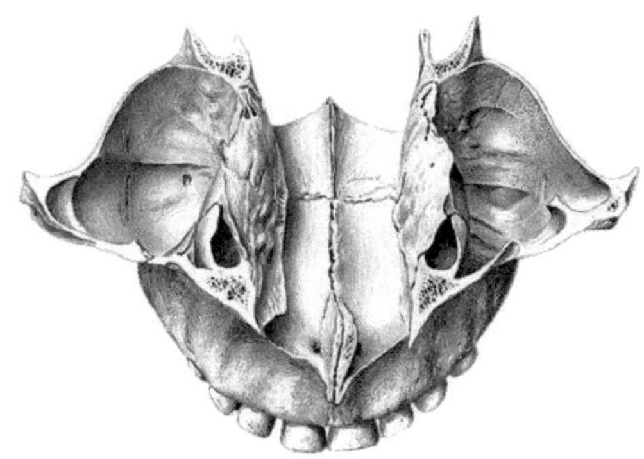

Figure 15*Axial section of the maxillary sinus.* [39]

- Vascularization and innervation :

Arteries come mainly from the middle meatus arteries and branches of the maxilla, with the venous network draining into the spheno-palatine vein and pterygoid plexus.

The innervation is provided by the trigeminal-sympathetic system of the nasal cavities and the nerves of the superior alveolar and infraorbital nerves.

3.1.2.3 The frontal sinus :

These are two pneumatic, asymmetrical cavities carved into the thickness of the frontal bone, communicating with the nasal fossae via the nasofrontal canal. The frontal sinus is shaped like a triangular pyramid with :

- An anterior or cutaneous wall, convex in front, connected to the cutaneous and subcutaneous planes, supraorbital and supratrochlear arteries, sensory nerves branches of V and motor nerves branches of VII, veins and lymphatics.

- A posterior or cerebral wall, connected to the meninges and frontal lobe.

- An inferior or orbito-nasal wall, the floor of the frontal region, with a medial nasal segment and a lateral orbital segment, forming the anteromedial part of the orbital vault, in contact with the orbital contents,

- A medial or inter-sinusal wall: a compact, thin, fragile, anteroposterior layer of bone separating the two frontal sinuses.

- The nasofrontal canal ensures drainage and ventilation of the frontal sinus, connecting it with the corresponding nasal cavity, which varies in shape and length according to the degree of development of the anterior ethmoidal cells, through which it travels, ending at the upper end of the uncibullar gutter.

- Vascularization and innervation are provided by the anterior ethmoidal artery and the arteries of the middle meatus, the trigemino-sympathetic system of the nasal cavities, and branches of the ophthalmic nerve.

3.1.2.4 The sphenoidal sinus :

This is the deepest cavity of the sinus complex. It follows Onodi's cell (the ethmoid-fronto-sphenoidal cell). It is even and median, housed in the cancellous bone of the sphenoid body. It is the only cavity that drains outside the ethmoidal meatus systems, opening directly into the posterosuperior wall of the corresponding nasal cavity (**Figure 16**).

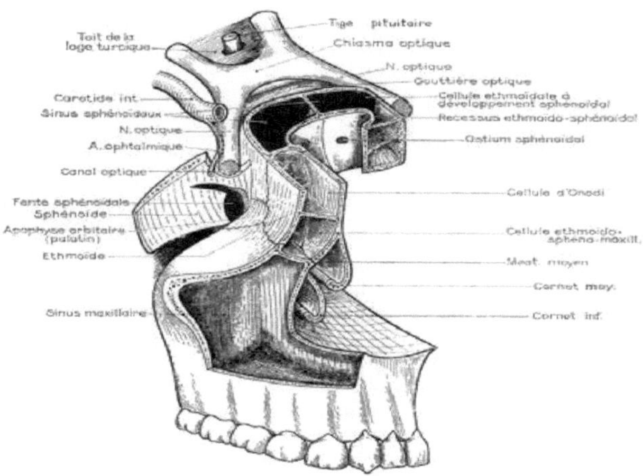

Figure 16*Sphenoid sinus ratio and drainage route (after Perlemuter & Legent).* [14]

Each sinus has six walls:

- The anterior or nasal wall:

The wall, which is surgically accessed, responds mainly in its lateral portion to the posterior ethmoidal cells, and in its medial segment to the nasal cavity, forming the spheno-ethmoidal recess, seat of the sphenoidal ostium.

- The bottom wall or floor :

This thick structure forms the upper wall of the nasopharyngeal cavum. Reinforced by the lower sphenoidal ridge, the spread of the two vomerian wings and the lateral pterygoid process. The three vomerovaginal ducts, the two pterygoid or vidian ducts, and the two palato-vaginal ducts run from inside to outside.

- The top wall or roof :

It responds to the anterior and middle layers of the skull, from which it is separated by the dura mater. This wall is divided into the sphenoidal jugum (olfactory region), the optic region and the saddle turcica (pituitary region).

It responds medially to the meninges, olfactory tract, optic chiasm and pituitary gland.

- Posterior wall :

It faces the posterior part of the skull, from which it is separated by a lamina of spongy bone tissue and dura mater, through which it responds to the basilar trunk, which bifurcates into the posterior cerebral arteries, the two VI nerves, and the bridge.

- The lateral wall or ophthalmic wall:

Thin wall connected from back to front with the cavernous sinus cavity, containing the internal carotid artery, the nerves of the orbital fissure (VI, III, IV and ophthalmic), the maxillary nerve, and the optic canal containing the optic nerve and ophthalmic artery, the posterior end of the medial wall of the orbit and the medial end of the superior orbital fissure.

- The medial wall or inter-sinus partition:

Inconsistent, sometimes dehiscent, it separates the two sphenoidal sinuses into two cavities, most often asymmetrical.

- Vascularization and innervation :

Provided by the ostial artery, branch of the naso-palatine artery, transosseous arteries, branches of the internal carotid artery, pterygoid canal and palato-vaginal canal.

Innervation depends on the trigeminal-sympathetic system of the nasal cavities and the posterior ethmoidal nerve.

3.2 Endonasal anatomy : [39,42,44-46]

A good knowledge of nasal and sinus anatomy is essential before embarking on endonasal endoscopy. Using a 0° or 30° endoscope, examination of the nasal cavity involves three essential steps:

-The first pass of the endoscope is used to locate the various anatomical elements of the nasal cavity: nasal valve, septum, inferior turbinate, middle turbinate and choana. It also enables the identification of any variations or modifications to the normal anatomy that may interfere with the surgical procedure. (**Figure 17**)

-the second pass examines the middle meatus from front to back: head of the middle turbinate, unciform process, ethmoidal bulla, retrobullary groove. The spheno-ethmoidal recess is then examined, revealing the sphenoidal ostium (**Figure 18**).

-the third pass allows examination of the ethmoidal infundibulum, while following the unciform process and the ethmoidal bulla, drainage orifices can be visualized.

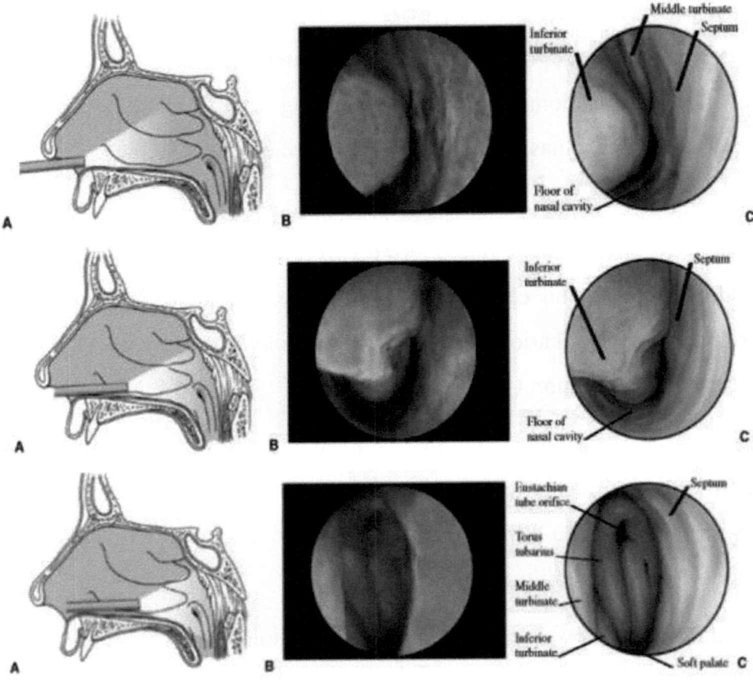

Figure 17*First passage of the endoscope.* [39]

3.2.1 Cones:

3.2.1.1 Lower horn :

This is the first structure visible when the endoscope is inserted, consisting of a head, body and tail. Its head is located about 1cm behind the piriform orifice.

The lower horn averages 45 mm in length. Its tail is part of the lateral wall of the choana.

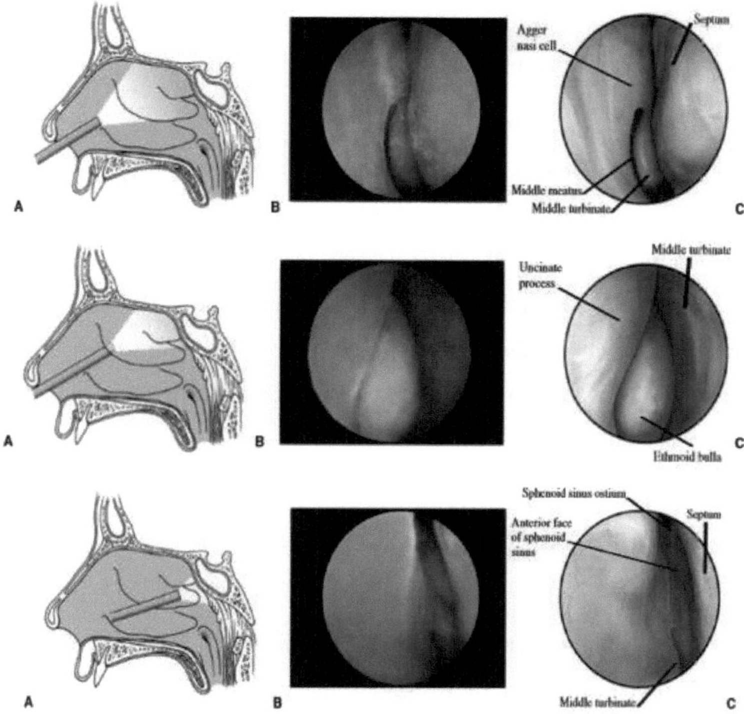

Figure 18*Middle and posterior view of the endoscope*. [39]

3.2.1.2 Medium horn :

By far the most important landmark in the nasal cavity, it lies above and behind the lower turbinate, which consists of a head, body and tail.

Measuring 40 mm in length, its usual curvature is concave medially, but it is subject to numerous physiological variations: pneumatization, paradoxical convexity. Its tail forms the lateral wall of the spheno-ethmoidal recess.

3.2.1.3 Upper horn :

It is difficult to see, often requiring the endoscope to be biased upwards in order to examine it; it is located above and behind the middle turbinate.

Its average length is 17 mm. The posterior part of its free edge lies a few millimeters outside the ostium of the sphenoidal sinus.

3.2.2 The meatic region:

3.2.2.1 Lower meatus :

The anterior end of the meatus is formed by the head of the inferior turbinate medially, and the lateral wall represented by the maxillary process laterally. The endoscope is slid along the floor of the nasal cavity, then moved backwards and forwards. Careful examination in the anterosuperior quadrant reveals the lower orifice of the nasolacrimal duct, aided by the flow of tears.

3.2.2.2 Middle meatus :

Its medial wall is formed by the middle turbinate, and its lateral wall by the three reliefs of the nasal wall of the ethmoidal labyrinth.

The lacrimal hump corresponds to the nasolacrimal duct, which is an anterior curve just in front of the head of the middle turbinate. Just behind it, a depression between the lacrimal bump and the unciform process, then comes the relief of the unciform process behind.

The unciform process originates opposite the anterior attachment of the head of the middle horn on the lateral wall, then descends vertically for about two centimetres, heading horizontally backwards.

The third relief is the anterior bullar wall, masked laterally by the relief of the unciform process. The depression of the semilunar hiatus or uncibullar gutter is formed by these two reliefs; at its upper end (ethmoidal infundibulum) is the gutter star or bullar traffic circle, and at its lower end is the ostium of the maxillary sinus.

3.2.2.3 Upper meatus :

Its medial wall is formed by the superior horn, which forms the lateral wall of the spheno-ethmoidal recess. The posterior ethmoidal cells drain into this meatus.

3.2.3 Spheno-ethmoidal recess:

The spheno-ethmoidal recess is the most posterior and deepest region of the nasal cavity (**Figure 19**). It has a limited oval shape:

- Outside: through the tail of the middle horn and the free portion of the upper horn.

- Inward: through the nasal septum.

- Bottom: through the upper part of the choana.

- Back: through the medial part of the anterior surface of the sphenoidal sinus.

The ostium of the sphenoidal sinus, located in its anterior wall, allows drainage of this sinus, and is usually about one centimeter above the choanal arch.

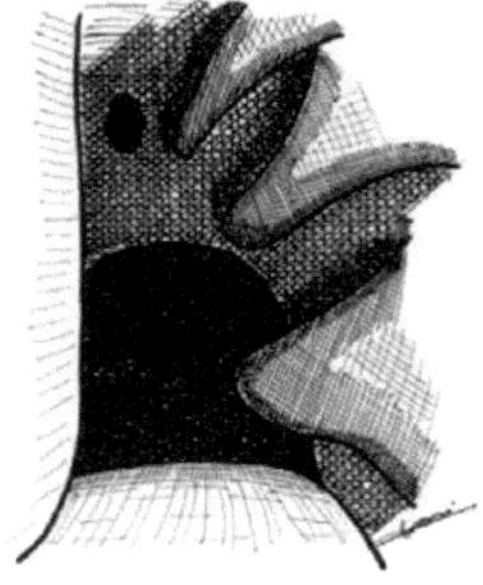

Figure 19*Left sphenoethmoidal ostium and recess*. [39]

3.2.4 The olfactory slit :

It's a narrowed space located between the upper part of the septum medially, and the upper attachment of the middle turbinate laterally.

3.3 Radiological anatomy : [39, 47,48]

3.3.1 Imaging technique:

3.3.1.1 Standard radiography :

The only really useful images for exploring the sinus cavities of the face are the Blondeau and ortho-pan-tomography.

The Blondeau incidence provides a global view of the facial mass, with the maxillary sinuses particularly well exposed. The nose and chin are located against the plate.

The upper edge of the boulders must lie below the alveolar recesses of the maxillary sinuses.

High frontal incidence provides a front view of the skull and facial mass. The upper edge of the boulders lies in the lower third of the orbits.

The ortho-pan-tomography or panoramic is a very important image that best explores the dental roots and any sinus teeth.

On the whole, standard x-rays provide limited information. They are currently neglected for two main reasons: firstly, the diagnosis of acute or chronic sinusitis is clinical; secondly, the poor quality of information provided by standard radiography often necessitates the use of CT scans.

3.3.1.2 Computed tomography (CT) :

This is the gold standard for exploring nasosinus cavities. The slice interval varies between 1 and 5 mm, depending on the indication and the number of planes to be performed. Intravenous injection of iodinated contrast is reserved for the study of tumoral lesions and complications of inflammatory rhinosinus pathology.

Virtual imaging is based on the same principle as static 3D acquisition. Dynamic approach software is used to "circulate" through the nasal cavity and the various sinus cavities along the drainage axes, providing access to small anatomical structures. This technique is particularly interesting for the surgeon, given the existence of multiple anatomical variants that can expose the surgeon to the risk of complications during endonasal surgery under endoscopic guidance.

3.3.1.3 Magnetic resonance imaging (MRI):

Cuts of 3 mm or less are required. 512x512 or 512x256 matrices give better resolution. Slice spacing is 2 to 5 mm, depending on the pathology studied. Standard sequences are T1-weighted and T2 spin echo. Gadolinium injection is useful for exploring inflammatory or tumoral pathologies.

3.3.2 Results:

3.3.2.1 Plan axial :

The lower sections pass through the floor of the maxillary sinus with the dental apices of the upper teeth, then highlight the anterolateral, posterior wall of the maxillary sinus, and the pterygopalatine fissure. The middle turbinate closes the ostium of the maxillary sinus. The nasal septum can be seen on the midline. Successive horizontal sections, moving cranially upwards, reveal the ethmoidal labyrinth above the maxillary sinus.

The median axial section shows the partitioning root of the middle turbinate. Axial sections show the sphenoidal sinus behind the posterior ethmoid, and the frontal sinus above the anterior ethmoid (**Figure 20**).

3.3.2.2 Coronal plane :

Coronal sections are particularly interesting for highlighting the different meatus of the nasal cavities with the turbinates. They enable visualization of the relationship between the medial wall of the maxillary sinus and the nasal cavities, and the relationship between the optic nerve and the sphenoidal sinus (**Figure 20**).

3.3.2.3 Sagittal plane :

Sagittal sections allow analysis of the systematization of the ethmoid, and the relationship of the nasofrontal canal with the anterior cells. They show the relationship of the sphenoid to the pituitary fossa (**Figure 20**).

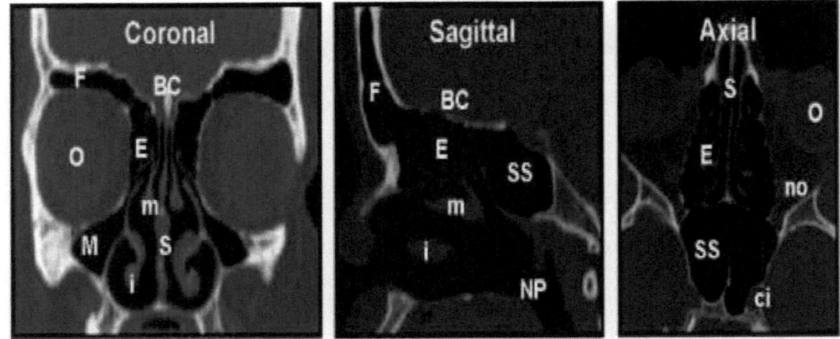

Figure 20*CT scan of the facial mass in a patient with no rhinosinus pathology: coronal, sagittal and axial sections* [49]

(BC: skull base; ci: internal carotid artery; E: ethmoidal sinus; F: frontal sinus; i: inferior turbinate; M: maxillary sinus; m: middle turbinate; no: optic nerve; NP: nasopharynx; O: orbit; S: nasal septum; SS: sphenoidal sinus).

References :

[11] Mahassine EL HARRAS, "la polypose nasosinusienne: place de la chirurgie endonasale", Université CADI AYYAD, Marrakech, 2011.

[14] F. Legent, L. Perlemuter, Cl. Vandenbrouck, *Cahiers d'anatomie ORL*, 4e ed., vol. 2. Masson, 1986.

[15] SOULTANA RABIE, "nasosinusal polyposis: experience of the ENT department at Moulay Ismail Hospital in Meknes (à propos de 60 cas)", Université Sidi Mohammed ben Abdellah, FES, 2015.

[33] E. Masson, "Anatomy of the nasosinus cavities," *EM-Consulte.* https://www.em-consulte.com/article/1139319/anatomie-des-cavites-nasosinusiennes (accessed Feb. 27, 2019).

[34] P. Kamina and C. Martinet, *Anatomie clinique : Tome 2, Tête, cou, dos*, 4e édition. Maloine, 2013.

[35] Rouvière and Delmas, *Anatomie humaine descriptive topographique et fonctionnelle, tome 1 : Tête et cou*, 15th ed. Paris: Editions Masson, 2002.

[36] A. Lahlaïdi, *Anatomie topographique: Applications anatomo-chirurgicales,*. Rabat: Livres Ibn Sina, 1986.

[37] L. Dialogues, *Gray's Anatomy for Students - Jacques Duparc, Fabrice Duparc, A. Mitchell, A.... - Elsevier Masson.* .

[38] R. L. (1950-) Drake *et al*, *Gray's atlas of human anatomy / Richard L. Drake, A. Wayne Vogl, Adam W. M. Mitchell, Richard M. Tibbitts, Paul E. Richardson*. Elsevier-Masson. Issy-les-Moulineaux, 2017.

[39] H. Levine and M. P. Clemente, *Sinus Surgery: Endoscopic and Microscopic Approaches*. Thieme, 2005.

[40] D. W. Hsu and J. D. Suh, "Anatomy and Physiology of Nasal Obstruction," *Otolaryngol. Clin. North Am.* vol. 51, n° 5, pp. 853-865, Oct. 2018, doi: 10.1016/j.otc.2018.05.001.

[41] S. M. Lieberman, "Anatomical landmarks in revision sinus surgery and advanced nasal polyposis," *Oper. Tech. Otolaryngol.-Head Neck Surg.* vol. 25, n° 2, pp. 149-155, June 2014, doi: 10.1016/j.otot.2014.02.003.

[42] R. Bradoo, *Anatomical Principles of Endoscopic Sinus Surgery: A Step by Step Approach*, 1 edition. London u.a.: CRC Press, 2005.

[43] A. Fatakia, R. Winters, and R. G. Amedee, "Epistaxis: A Common Problem," *Ochsner J.*, vol. 10, n° 3, pp. 176-178, 2010.

[44] klossek J-M, Serrano E, Dessi P, Fontanel J-P, "Chirurgie endonasale sous guidage endoscopique", 3rd Edition, Masson, 2004.

[45] J.-M. Klossek and C. B. de Montreuil, *Chirurgie du nez, des fosses nasales et des sinus*. Issy-les-Moulineaux: Elsevier Masson, 2007.

[46] F. Facon and P. Dessi, "Microinvasive endonasal surgery: contribution of endoscopy in maxillofacial surgery",

/data/revues/00351768/01060004/230/, Feb. 2008, Accessed: March 20, 2019. [Online]. Available from: https://www.em-consulte.com/en/article/94856.

[47] " Radioanatomy of the facial sinuses - EM|consult". https://www.em-consulte.com/en/article/121593 (accessed March 20, 2019).

[48] Vivarrat-Perrin L, Veillon F, "Radioanatomie du crâne, du rocher, de l'orbite, des sinus, de la mandibule et des dents." mars 01, 2019, [Online]. Available from: http://www.med.univ.

[49] P. Champsaur, T. Pascal, V. Vidal, J. Gaubert, J. Bartoli, and G. Moulin, "Radioanatomy of the facial sinuses," p. 16, 2019.

Chapitre 4 : Histological review: [14,15,50-52]

The bony relief of the nasal cavity is softened by the nasal or pituitary mucosa, which rests on the periosteum and perichondrium that line the bony and cartilaginous walls. This nasal mucosa continues with the mucosa of the sinuses and the nasolacrimal duct.

It is made up of a chorion and an epithelium that varies according to the region of the nasal cavity: vestibular region, olfactory region and respiratory region.

4.1 Vestibular region :

The entrance to the nasal cavity is covered by cutaneous tissue. A transition zone between skin and respiratory mucosa lies behind this vestibular region, extending to the head of the middle and lower turbinates. It is characterized by an epidermis that has lost its stratum corneum and glands, usually present in the skin.

4.2 Olfactory region :

This region is represented by the olfactory fossa, which forms the upper part of the nasal cavity. It lies above the olfactory cleft, bounded by the lower edge of the middle turbinate, on the outside, and the tubercle of the septum, on the inside.

4.2.1 Macroscopic appearance :

The mucous membrane is smooth, yellow or brownish, hence the name locus luteus, with a thickness of around one and a half millimeters.

4.2.2 Microscopic appearance :

- **Epithelium:** cylindrical, stratified, comprising :

- Schultze's olfacto-sensory cells are spindle-shaped and bipolar, with a peripheral extension flush with the surface and terminating in a hemispherical bulge covered with short, rigid olfactory cilia. Another central extension crosses the chorion to reach the olfactory bulb.

- Support cells, which occupy the entire height of the epithelium. They support the sensory cells they surround. They are cylindrical in shape, with a granular cytoplasm containing the yellow pigment.

- The basal cells, which are small, irregular and star-shaped, form a single layer lying deep down on the chorion.

- **Chorion:** characterized by the presence of voluminous tubuloacinar glands called Bowman's glands, open at the surface by a small pertus. The glandular cells, of uncertain nature, also contain a yellow pigment.

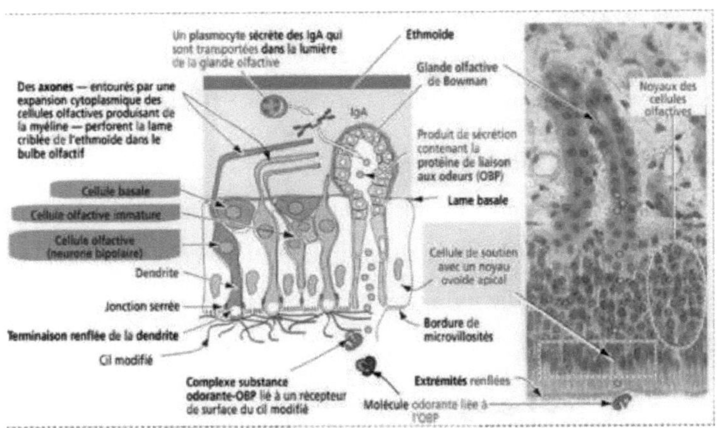

Figure 21*Olfactory epithelium.* [51]

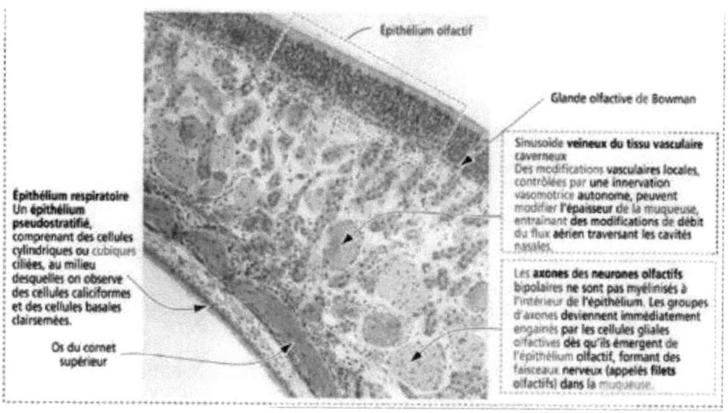

Figure 22*Olfactory mucosa.* [51]

4.3 Respiratory region :

The respiratory mucosa occupies the largest part, with a surface area of around 75 cm^3 . There is a gradual transition to the vestibular mucosa and an abrupt one to the olfactory mucosa.

4.3.1 Macroscopic appearance :

Bright red in color, about 2 to 3 mm thick.

4.3.2 Microscopic appearance :

- **Epithelium:** surface, respiratory-type, pseudostratified, prismatic and ciliated. The composition of this epithelium varies throughout the airways, depending on the anatomical region; at least seven main cell types can be identified:

- ciliated cells, found mainly in the respiratory mucosa, prismatic in shape, elongated, resting on the basement membrane and covered at the apical end with vibratory cilia.

- the muciparous or caliciform cells, located between the ciliated cells, but varying in number from region to region. They are particularly numerous in exposed areas such as the heads of the turbinates. In some areas, they form small clusters, forming intra-epithelial glands. They seem to originate from the transformation of ciliated cells.

- undifferentiated intermediate cells, involved in epithelial regeneration.

- serous cells, mainly found in sub-epithelial glands.

- brush cells, involved in hydroelectrolytic exchange.

- rare neuroendocrine cells, secreting neuropeptides.

- basal cells, which are small, triangular cells that form a single layer on top of the basal membrane.

This respiratory epithelium rests on a thin basement membrane, which separates it from the underlying chorion. It is absent from the olfactory region.

- Chorion: conjunctivo-elastic density varies from region to region, with elastic elements predominating in the turbinates. Its main feature is the presence of compound glands, especially in the middle part, with glandular cells arranged in a single layer continuing the epithelial layer and including mucous cells and serous cells. It is also characterized by its wealth of vascular elements, particularly venous, lymphatic and nerve. The presence of so-called "motile" cells, such as isolated lymphocytes or lymphocytes organized in clusters (nose associated lymphoid tissue, NALT) [9,10].

In the face of airborne contaminants, the nasal epithelium forms a physical and functional barrier, thanks to junction complexes. Epithelial cells are linked apically by tight junctions and laterally by desmosomes, which maintain epithelial integrity and form a physical barrier. Breaking the integrity of this epithelial barrier directly exposes the underlying cells to toxic agents in the air. The cells thus stimulated can initiate an inflammatory reaction.

4.4 Mucous membrane of the facial sinuses :

The mucosa of the sinus cavities adjoining the nasal cavities is of the same respiratory type. It is considered an extension of the nasal mucosa, with the distinctive feature of being much less vascularized, thinner and more fragile. The mucosa comprises an epithelium, a basement membrane and a chorion.

4.4.1 Epithelium:

The epithelium is respiratory, cylindrical, stratified and ciliated. It contains four cell types, all in intimate contact with the basement membrane. Epithelial cells include :

- **basal cells:** these are replacement cells linked to the basal membrane by means of receptors called "integrins". As they multiply, they give rise to daughter cells that can regenerate the other three cell types;

- **caliciform cells:** they manufacture, store and excrete mucins, an important component of mucus. Once they have expelled their contents, they take on the shape of a calyx. By invaginating into the chorion, they form tubuloacinar glands.

- **cells with microvilli:** microvilli increase cell surface area. These cells are rich in mitochondria and smooth endoplasmic reticulum. They have intense metabolic activity. They are involved in transepithelial fluid exchange, and in maintaining and renewing the periciliary aqueous film.

- **hair cells:** represent nearly 80% of the cell population.

4.4.2 The chorion or lamina propria :

It contains an extracellular matrix of collagen fibers, vessels, seromucous glands and inflammatory cells. Deep down, the connective tissue condenses into a true periosteum, in continuity with the chorion. It comprises three layers:

- **the subepithelial layer:** rich in lymphocytes, plasma cells, histiocytes and macrophages.

- **the glandular layer:** contains tubuloacinar seromucous glands surrounded by myoepithelial cells. They arise from invagination of the caliciform cells of the epithelium and participate in mucus production with the epithelial cells. They are smaller and less numerous than in the nasal cavities, and more abundant in the vicinity of the sinus ostium. A distinction is made between mucous cells and serous cells. Mucous cells contain mucins and immunoglobulins (Ig) A . Serous cells synthesize glycoproteins, antibacterial proteins (lactoferrin, lysozyme) and antioxidants (transferrin and anti-leukoproteases).

- **the vascular layer:** formed by a network of fenestrated sub-epithelial capillaries connected to arteriovenous anastomoses in the deep chorion. Unlike the nasal cavities, there are no capacitance vessels.

References :

[9] Peynegre, Freche, Fontanel, *la polypose naso sinusienne*. Société Française d'Oto-rhino-laryngologie et de Chirurgie de la Face et du Cou, 2000.

[10] T. M. Önerci and B. J. Ferguson, eds, *Nasal Polyposis: Pathogenesis, Medical and Surgical Treatment*. Berlin Heidelberg: Springer-Verlag, 2010.

[14] F. Legent, L. Perlemuter, Cl. Vandenbrouck, *Cahiers d'anatomie ORL*, 4e ed., vol. 2. Masson, 1986.

[15] SOULTANA RABIE, "nasosinusal polyposis: experience of the ENT department at Moulay Ismail Hospital in Meknes (à propos de 60 cas)", Université Sidi Mohammed ben Abdellah, FES, 2015.

[50] B. Young, G. O'Dowd, and P. Woodford, *Wheater's atlas of functional histology*. De Boeck supérieur, 2015.

[51] W. Kühnel and B. Samama, *Atlas de poche d'histologie*, 5th ed. Paris: Médecine Sciences Publications, 2015.

[52] A. L. Kierszenbaum, P. Validire, and P. Validire-Charpy, *Histology and cell biology: An introduction to pathological anatomy*. Brussels: De Boeck, 2015.

Chapitre 5 : Physiology of the nasosinus cavities : [29,39,53-55]

5.1 Physiology of the nasal cavity :

The nasal cavities, which form part of the airways as a whole, are not inert ducts. Their role is to shape the aerodynamic and physico-chemical characteristics of the air breathed in. They are recognized for :

- Respiratory function (nasal resistance, shape, direction, volume and velocity of airflow): The nasal cycle (regulated by the vegetative, sympathetic and parasympathetic nervous systems) allows an alternation of decongestion between the right and left sides every 3 or 4 hours.

- Conditioning function by heating and humidifying inspired air.

- Filtration by the mucociliary carpet.

- Phonation (sound box).

- Olfaction.

5.1.1 Airflow control :

During inspiration, thoracic depression creates a negative intrathoracic pressure that draws air through the nasal cavities, whose internal morphology regulates the shape, direction and flow of air passing through them.

The characteristic of air traffic in the nasal cavity, with its abrupt back-and-forth movements of density over a turbulent, viscous wall, gives rise to a turbulent, continuously unstable regime.

5.1.2 Filter and purification function:

The swirling movements of the airflow created by the tormented architecture of the nasal cavity promote contact between the inspired air volume and the nasal mucosa.

A large proportion of the particles inhaled then collide with the mucus, where they remain trapped. They are then expelled by the mucociliary movement.

5.1.3 Humidification :

The essential mechanisms for understanding the transfer of water from the 95% water-containing mucus to the inspired air stream are convection and diffusion.

The network of subepithelial fenestrated capillaries seems to play a fundamental role in the regulation and rapid adaptation of water exchange. The renal filtration-reabsorption-like regulation system of microvilli cells would complete this regulation.

5.1.4 Warming :

The 37°C blood circulating in the central vessels constantly passes through the arteriovenous shunts present in the deep chorion, warming the nasal cavity like a central heating system.

5.1.5 Immune function :

A function organized in three lines:

- first line of epithelial defense, through the epithelial barrier formed by the cellular arrangement placed on a basal membrane acting as a filter for molecules and the muco-ciliary system thanks to lytic enzymes and secretory IgA.

This mucociliary purification is a fundamental element in the defense of the airways in general. Its dysfunction, as in cystic fibrosis or ciliary dyskinesia, predisposes to the development of chronic infectious and inflammatory processes in the rhinosinus apparatus. [56].

- second specific line of defense: the immune system annexed to the nasal mucosa, through secretory IgA and other immune system components;

playing the role of inhibiting bacterial adhesion to the mucosal surface, neutralizing viruses and toxins and preventing antigen absorption.

- third line of defense: nonspecific inflammation, which is continually called upon by inflammation factors due to the nasal mucosa's frontline position in the respiratory tract.

5.1.6 Olfactory function :

To stimulate the olfactory nerve receptors in the nasal cavity, odorant molecules carried in the inspired air must pass through the olfactory cleft region. Highly situated, this passage is facilitated by the congested state of the lower turbinates during the nasal cycle.

5.2 Sinus physiology:

The paranasal sinuses are aerial cavities hollowed out of the skull bones. They appear as physiologically silent cavities, whose homeostasis is governed by the properties of their mucous membrane, made up of a respiratory-type epithelium, cylindrically ciliated pseudostratified; involved in gas exchange. And the ostia, which communicate with the nasal fossae.

These ostia are the obligatory passageway for air, and the point of convergence for the various drainage pathways. The permeability of this orifice and the proper functioning of the mucociliary drainage activity are crucial to maintaining sinus physiology.

5.2.1 Physiology of the sinus mucosa :

- **Conditioning function :**

The sinus mucosa is endowed with the property of absorbing oxygen and rejecting carbon dioxide, and in addition to its secretion capacity, it has reabsorption capabilities. These mechanisms can play an important role in chronic ostial obstruction.

- **Immune function :**

Physiologically, the intra-sinus environment is sterile. Morphologically, the three lines of defense specific to the respiratory mucosa are present.

But with a clear predominance of the first line of epithelial defense, represented by the mucociliary carpet of the sinus mucosa.

Mucus contains :

-Mucins, present in the viscous surface layer of mucus, neutralize microorganisms.

- Lysozymes, secreted by serous cells. They have bacteriolytic activity and stimulate the phagocytic activity of leukocytes and macrophages.

- IgA is synthesized by submucosal plasma cells. They are excreted by the seromucosal glands. They inhibit bacterial adhesion to the epithelium, neutralize viruses in the cells and promote the phagocytic activity of inflammatory cells.

- Transferrin, secreted by serous cells. It binds the iron needed for bacterial growth.

- Antioxidants (transferrin and anti-leukoproteases) to combat free radicals from toxic products or inflammatory cells.

- **Role of nitric oxide (NO) :**

This highly reactive free radical is produced in large quantities in the sinuses. The enzymes responsible for its production (NO synthetases) are present in the cilia and microvilli of the epithelium.

It contributes to sinus sterility thanks to its antibacterial and antiviral properties and its action on ciliary activity. It is also a marker of inflammation.

In adulthood, the sinus mucosa continuously produces NO, which is actively released into the inspired air and transported to the pulmonary alveoli, where it increases arterial blood oxygenation.

Its concentration in nasal exhaled air decreases in pathologies where the sinuses are filled with mucus or the ostia are blocked, as in the case of nasosinus polyposis.

- **Tissue defense mechanisms :**

They take place in the lamina propria of the sinus mucosa. The chorion is rich in mononuclear elements: monocytes, macrophages, lymphocytes and plasma cells. All these cellular elements belong to the NALT or lymphoid tissue associated with the nasosinus mucosa.

This is where IgA and secretory IgA are secreted into the mucus. It also contains T-helper lymphocytes.

5.2.2 Physiology of the ostium :

The ostium represents a transition zone between the nasal and sinus mucosa, protecting the sinus and helping to maintain intra-sinus physiological constants.

Trans-ostial sinus ventilation ensures continuous renewal of intra-sinus air and compensates for transmucosal gas exchange.

- **Intra-sinus air:**

Its composition differs from that of inspiratory and expiratory air, with 2.2% CO_2 and 17.5% O_2 . It is 2°C cooler than body temperature and has a high humidity level, reaching 100%. Intra-sinus pressure, on the other hand, is in equilibrium with atmospheric pressure, with variations depending on the context (physical exertion or nose blowing increases pressure, sniffing decreases it).

- **Transmucosal gas exchange :**

Air in the sinus comes from trans-ostial and trans-epithelial gas exchange. Gas exchange through the ostium is mainly by diffusion.

The sinus mucosa is permeable to gases, enabling exchanges between the sinus cavity and the blood that irrigates it. In the absence of sinus air renewal, transepithelial gas exchange tends to maintain equilibrium.

Obstruction of the ostium leads to a decrease in oxygen partial pressure and an increase in CO2 partial pressure. Ciliary activity diminishes, and mucus stagnates. Secondary bacterial proliferation and inflammatory hypertrophy of the mucosa increase ostial obstruction.

References :

[29] R. Jankowski, *Du dysfonctionnement naso-sinusien chronique au dysfonctionnement ostio-meatal.* Paris: Société Française d'Oto-rhino-laryngologie et de Chrurgie de la Face et du Cou, 2006.

[39] H. Levine and M. P. Clemente, *Sinus Surgery: Endoscopic and Microscopic Approaches*. Thieme, 2005.

[53] R. Jankowski and C. Rumeau, "Physiology of the ostium of the paranasal sinuses: endoscopic observations", *Ann. Fr. Oto-Rhino-Laryngol. Pathol. Cervico-Faciale*, vol. 135, n° 2, pp. 144-145, Apr. 2018, doi: 10.1016/j.aforl.2017.09.005.

[54] E. Masson, "Physiology of the paranasal sinuses", *EM-Consulte.* https://www.em-consulte.com/article/30716/physiologie-des-sinus-paranasaux (accessed March 26, 2019).

[55] J. M. Klossek, "La physiologie naso-sinusienne", *Rev. Fr. Allergol. Immunol. Clin*, vol. 38, n° 7, pp. 579-583, Jan. 1998, doi: 10.1016/S0335-7457(98)80121-4.

[56] A. Wanner, M. Salathé, and T. G. O'Riordan, "Mucociliary clearance in the airways," *Am. J. Respir. Crit. Care Med.* vol. 154, n° 6 Pt 1, pp. 1868-1902, Dec. 1996, doi: 10.1164/ajrccm.154.6.8970383.

Chapitre 6 : Etiopathogenesis

6.1 Epidemiology :

6.1.1 Frequency:

The prevalence of SNP in the general population has been roughly estimated at between 1 and 4%, although the multiplicity of definitions suggests an overestimation of SNP [2,57,58].

Earlier reports suggested a prevalence ranging from 0.2 [59] à 2,2% [60]and autopsy studies have reported an incidence of bilateral PNS ranging from 1.5 [61] à 2% [4].

6.1.2 Age :

It has been suggested that the incidence of SNP increases with age. Settipane [62] reported that its frequency peaks in patients aged 50 and over. Furthermore, he reports that asthmatics over 40 are four times more likely to have SFN than those under 40 (12.4 vs. 3.1%, $p < 0.01$).

Larsen et al [57] reported similar results in a uniform population of Danish patients. Out of 252 patients, they observed PNS most frequently in patients aged between 40 and 60. Moreover, its presence in patients over 80 years of age was unlikely. The mean age at diagnosis of PNS was 51 for men and 49 for women.

The discovery of PNS in children is extremely rare. Its incidence in patients under 16 years of age ranges from 0.1 [62] and 0.216% [57].

6.1.3 Gender :

As with age, the literature varies on the impact of gender on the development of SNP. Settipane [63] examining 211 patients with SNP, found an equal distribution of men and women, 50.2% versus 49.8% respectively.

More recently, based on the Danish national health insurance system, Larsen et al. [57] identifying patients treated for SNP, this cohort showed an increased incidence of SNP in men over 20 compared with women of the same age. The male/female ratio of patients with SNP was 2.9 in the 40-50 age group, and a maximum of 6.0 in patients aged 80-89.

Incidence was equally high in men and women aged 40 to 69. In this group, PNS was present in 1.68 men and 0.82 women per thousand per year [57].

6.1.4 Contributing factors :

Various comorbidities such as allergic rhinitis, generalized atopic status and asthma have all been proposed as incriminating factors in the genesis of SFN. However, the data for these associations have been the subject of ongoing investigations and discrepancies between authors. Variations in prevalence have also been reported as a function of demographic factors, including age and gender. In addition, hereditary factors and ethnic variations exist and need to be taken into account.

6.1.4.1 Environmental factors :

Certain environmental factors can influence SFN, including climate, pollution, smoking and allergens. Although some patients report improvement or worsening due to climatic factors, the latter appear to play a negligible role.

There are no data on the role of climatic factors in the literature, probably due to the negligible role they play, as SFN is found in all climates and altitudes. Changes in the seasonal clinical expression of SFN are rarely observed.

The influence of pollution on allergic diseases and rhinitis has been the subject of a few studies, including a single French study on SFN [64]. This French multicenter prospective study, involving 224 patients, clarified the responsibility of environmental factors such as urban pollution. No significant difference was found between the incidence of SNP in rural and urban areas, so pollution does not appear to be a determining factor.

6.1.4.2 Allergy and asthma:

If, for a long time, from the era of Younge in 1907 [65]polyposis has often been considered an allergic disease, it is currently accepted that it is not associated with atopy. At most, in some patients, atopy may be considered an aggravating factor.

The increase in IgE found in some SNPs could be a consequence of polyposis and not a cause: for some, the existence in polyps of abraded epithelial surfaces would facilitate sensitization to pneumallergens [66]. Others question the very existence of this epithelial abrasion [65].

The late age of onset of SNP, the frequently intrinsic nature of the asthma sometimes associated with it, and the precession by a NARES in some cases, are not arguments in favour of the allergic hypothesis [65,67].

Furthermore, an allergic mechanism could only be considered as the main pathophysiological factor in a very small percentage of cases, such as allergic fungal sinusitis [68].

On the other hand, a number of current studies point to the role of microbial allergy in the genesis of certain SNPs. By measuring IgE antibodies specific to purified proteins extracted from 16 types of bacteria in the serum of patients with polyps, they conclude that IgE-dependent hypersensitivity may be caused by sensitization to sinus-infecting bacteria.

Even more recently, authors have attempted to distinguish between allergic and non-allergic SNPs, either by the difference in the inflammatory cells involved, or by the difference in the profile of cytokines secreted [69-71]. Classic publications have suggested that polyp formation is the product of an allergic reaction, due to a certain atopy through inhalation of allergens. Although this relationship seems intuitive, current data suggest that this association is weak.

The prevalence of SNP in patients with allergic rhinitis is estimated at 1.5 [63] and 1.7% [72]This rate approaches that of the general population.

Large cohort studies have shown a strong association between asthma and SFN, while the relationship between atopy and SFN has always been questioned. Settipane [62] in a survey of over 2,000 patients, reported that SFN was more frequent in non-allergic asthmatic patients, than in allergic asthmatic patients (13 vs. 5%, $p < 0.01$).

These data were corroborated by Grigoeras et al. [72]who analyzed 3,817 Greek patients with chronic rhinitis and asthma. Overall, the incidence of SFN in this population was 4.2%, and the prevalence of SFN was highest in non-allergic asthmatics than in allergic asthmatics (13 vs. 2.4%). There was an association between SFN and permanent perennial allergy, in contrast to seasonal allergy.

Other studies [73] have examined how factors such as SNP and atopy may correlate with CRS severity, as measured by CT.

In a group of 193 CRS patients, statistical analysis revealed that atopy was significantly more prevalent in the CRS subgroup without polyps (32.3%) compared to those with polyps (27.5%). Although the mean Lund-Mackay score was slightly higher in atopic than in non-atopic patients (14.2 vs. 12.3, $p = 0.05$). In contrast, the increase in radiological severity was observed in the CRS subgroup with polyps. Overall, these data suggest that the presence of polyps is not related to atopy, which is a better predictor of the radiological evolution of the disease.

A similar study [74] examined 106 patients in a nursing home, 49% of whom were atopic according to skin test titration. Overall, atopic and non-atopic patients showed no difference in the prevalence of SNP (38 vs. 37%).

However, the presence of asthma was an independent predictor for the existence of SFN, which was observed in 57.6% of asthmatics versus 25% of non-asthmatics (p = 0.0015). As before, the Lund-Mackay score was highest in non-atopic asthmatics, followed by atopic asthmatics, then non-asthmatics. As expected, this same score was highest in the SFN group, but it is important to note that this association proved independent of patients' atopic status.

In summary, these data indicate that asthmatic patients are more likely to have polyps than non-asthmatics.

Furthermore, the presence of asthma and polyps was each a significant predictor of disease severity as measured by the Lund-Mackay score. In contrast, atopy appears unrelated or perhaps weakly related to polyp growth or disease progression radiologically.

6.1.4.3 Genetic factor :

Genetic inheritance has been proposed as a possible etiological factor in SNP. Studies have suggested that up to 14% of patients with this condition have a family history of SFN [75].

In a report of twins with cortico-dependent asthma, only one showed aspirin intolerance and SFN, while the other did not manifest these phenotypic features [76].

To demonstrate family associations in SNP, a study (57) of 174 patients with SNP found that 25% of patients had a first-degree relative with SNP. Of 44 patients with Widal's triad, 36% had a first-degree relative with

SFN. In addition, 32% of patients with SFN also had asthma, and 30% had a first-degree relative with SFN.

Although a genetic predisposition to polyp formation is an important factor, there is no clear pattern of inheritance in the vast majority of cases of SNP [77].

6.1.4.4 Aspirin intolerance:

SNPs are frequently observed in patients intolerant to aspirin (acetylsalicylic acid) or non-steroidal anti-inflammatory drugs (NSAIDs) . In this subgroup of patients, these drugs induce an acute asthma attack within 30 to 90 minutes of ingestion [78].

This "triad" of symptoms (bronchial asthma, PNS and aspirin intolerance) is often referred to as Samter's triad, ASA-triad or Fernand Widal triad. In patients with this triad, aspirin is thought to induce an acute bronchial response associated with rhinorrhea and nasal obstruction [79].

Aspirin intolerance causing urticaria without bronchospasm is not associated with SFN. It is estimated that up to 50% of aspirin-intolerant patients have SFN, and 36% of patients with SFN may have some form of analgesic intolerance [62]. However, considering all patients undergoing endoscopic sinus surgery, including CRS with and without polyps; around 4.6% had Fernand Widal triad [80].

The constitution of a complete triad is probably achieved over time. Initially, patients may present with chronic rhinitis. Within 5 to 10 years, aspirin-induced asthma becomes apparent. Shortly thereafter, polyps become prominent [81].

Non-allergic rhinitis with eosinophilia (NARES) has been proposed as a precursor to the Fernand Widal triad. Polyp epithelial cells in Fernand Widal syndrome have been shown to exhibit basement membrane abnormalities and aspirin-induced generation of eicosanoids (by-products of arachidonic acid metabolism, including prostaglandins, thromboxanes and leukotrienes), ultimately leading to aspirin intolerance [82,83].

Polyposis in the Fernand Widal triad probably represents a unique case of severe inflammation. It is more recalcitrant to medical treatment or surgical intervention. Moreover, the response to surgery in patients with Fernand Widal syndrome is universally poor. They undergo around ten times as many surgical procedures as aspirin-tolerant patients. In addition, patients have a significantly higher rate of symptom recurrence (nasal obstruction, facial pain, posterior jetage and anosmia), polyp recurrence at 6 months' follow-up and no statistical improvement in FEV1 (forced expiratory volume in one second) [80,84].

6.1.4.5 Allergic fungal rhinosinusitis:

Classically, the diagnosis of allergic fungal rhinosinusitis (AFRS), is made when the following five criteria are present:

-type I hypersensitivity to mycotic Damatiae,

-presence of nasal polyps,

-nasosinusal CT scan reveals densifications with pseudocalcifications,

-mucin rich in eosinophils, aspergillary truffles and Charcot-Leyden crystals. But no deep fungal invasion of the sinus mucosa,

and fungus-positive sinus mucus sampling.

A patient suspected of having RSFA rarely presents all five criteria. However, the diagnosis can be made on the basis of clinical and intraoperative suspicion by observation of eosinophilic mucus and polyps. Staining for fungal elements in intraoperative biopsies has been shown to be inconsistent even in patients strongly suspected of having RSFA. [8585-87][

The incidence of RSFA has not been well established, but patient characteristics probably influence the manifestation of the disease. Approximately 5-10% of CRS patients with polyps have RSFA. 86,88][

It is typically a disease of young adults, with an average age of diagnosis of 22 [89] and 28 years [90]which is significantly lower than that observed in patients without RSFA. Studies have suggested an increased prevalence of RSFA in regions with a more humid climate.

Recent reports have suggested that low socioeconomic status may also play a role. At a tertiary medical center in South Carolina, a significant proportion of patients with RSFA (24.1%) were uninsured or Medicaid recipients, compared with 5.2% of patients with CRS with polyps without RSFA. In addition, a large proportion of the group with RSFA were African-American (61.1%) who resided in the County with a greater proportion in advanced poverty status [90].

6.1.4.6 Ethnic and geographical factors :

As the exact mechanism of polyp formation remains a subject of research, ethnic and geographic variations have emerged as a potential modifier of pathophysiology.

In a Caucasian population, polyps had a strong eosinophilic component, probably due to retrocontrol of interleukin (IL) -5 [91]. In addition to IL-5, eotaxin and eosinophil proteins are significantly elevated in polyp homogenate indicating amplification of eosinophilic inflammation [92].

In addition, the growth factor TGF-b1, a cytokine known to stimulate extracellular matrix and inhibit IL-5 synthesis, is down-regulated in polyps. Consequently, a cytokine cascade leading to IL-5 overproduction, with down-regulation of TGF-b1 , may potentiate the eosinophil response and have deleterious effects on the extracellular matrix simultaneously [92,93].

In Asian countries, the pattern is neutrophilic rather than eosinophilic. However, the clinical manifestation of PNS remains similar between Asians and Caucasians. [94]

Zhang et al [95] attempted to characterize the variations observed in Asian polyps. Samples of polyp tissue from 27 Chinese patients from Guangdong province in China were collected; most Asian patients had been treated with nasal steroids and antibiotics, some had received Chinese herbal medicines. The samples were compared with a group of Caucasian Belgian patients.

In the Chinese, the incidence of eosinophils in polyps was significantly lower ($p < 0.01$).

A Korean study [96] showed a similar preponderance of non-eosinophilic polyps. Of the 30 patients with SFN in the study, not only were 66.7% of cases non-eosinophilic, but also the thickness of the basement membrane of their polyps was found to be much thinner in the non-eosinophilic group versus the eosinophilic group (8.2 ± 3.5 vs. 13.9 ± 4.5 mm).

It has been found that [91] that 10 cases of Asian polyps contained IgE directed against Staphylococcus aureus enterotoxins (ESA) , which is consistent with previously reported data that one-third of Caucasians with SNP and asthma have IgE to ESA. As in Caucasian subjects, tissue IgE and IL-2R are elevated in Asian polyps. TGF-b1 was significantly down-regulated in Asian polyps compared with inferior horn controls. Furthermore, TGF-b1 was extremely low in SNP groups with IgE to ESA, suggesting a modulatory effect of staphylococcal enterotoxins. This finding has already been observed in Caucasians.

It's clear that the physiology of polyposis varies between Asians and Caucasians, yet there were only limited investigations of other ethnic minorities and racial backgrounds.

A collaboration between three otorhinolaryngology departments from different continents, Eritrea (Africa), China (Asia) and Switzerland (Europe) has attempted to better characterize the racial variation of polyps [96].

In this report, the African and Chinese participants received no preoperative steroids or antibiotics, whereas the Caucasians were treated preoperatively with Prednisolone 1 mg / kg / day for 5 days as well as Trimethoprim / Sulfamethoxazole for 10 days. Compared with Chinese and Caucasians, Africans presented a more progressive disease with extensive, ulcerated polyposis. Eosinophil density was also higher in polyps from African patients ($p < 0.001$) compared to Chinese and Caucasian polyps. There was no difference in eosinophil count between Chinese and Caucasians. Plasma cells and lymphocytes were abundant in Chinese and Caucasian polyps and scarce in African polyps. No difference was observed in mast cell counts for any group.

Unfortunately, the patients included in these analyses were not standardized with respect to preoperative treatments. The Caucasian cohort had been treated with preoperative steroids, which would probably have eliminated the presence of inflammatory mediators in polyp biopsies.

The main cause of these disparities is probably due to the different socio-economic situation between the study countries, resulting in significant variation in patient access to healthcare and probably affecting the molecular data. While polyps from Caucasian and Asian patients may show cellular and molecular differences, it is possible that polyps from African patients may also show variations in cellular and molecular profile.

6.2 Pathogenesis :

6.2.1 Introduction :

A growing body of evidence suggests that SNP is a clinical manifestation of a possible coexistence of multiple immunological factors.

The underlying mechanisms that contribute to the chronic nasal inflammation seen in SNP are not fully elucidated at present.

Various research groups have focused on exploring the role of nasosinus mucosal epithelial cells, the host immune system and pathogens in the pathogenesis of SFN. It is hypothesized that an impaired nasosinus epithelial barrier could lead to increased exposure to inhaled pathogens, antigens and particles which, in the case of a deregulated host immune response, could promote chronic inflammation [57,58,97].

Under normal, healthy conditions, the epithelial cells lining the nasal mucosa not only form a physical barrier to protect the host from inhaled pathogens and respiratory particles, but also play an essential role in mucociliary clearance and host immune defense. In CRS with polyps, the nasosinus epithelial barrier is defective, leading to increased tissue permeability, reduced epithelial resistance and destruction of the mucociliary carpet.

But why the epithelial barrier is defective in CRS with polyps remains unclear. It may be that the epithelial cells are intrinsically abnormal [98]. Alternatively, extrinsic factors specific to CRS with polyps could alter an otherwise intact epithelial barrier and induce the lesions observed in this case [99].

Other epithelial defense elements are also altered in CRS with polyps, leading to impaired mucociliary clearance, reduced secretion of antimicrobial defense proteins and degradation of the epithelial barrier.

These abnormalities can lead to chronic exposure to pathogenic and non-pathogenic molecules and the development of a chronic inflammatory response. [58]

Dysregulation of the host immune system has also been extensively evaluated in CRS with polyps. This disease was originally classified as a type 2 inflammatory response, with increased tissue eosinophilia.

Studies have also shown that CRS with polyps increases the number of basophils, lymphoid cells and mast cells. In addition, type 2 cytokines, including IL-5 and IL-13, as well as TSLP (thymic stroma derived from lymphopoietic epithelial cells) . While the inflammatory environment in CRS with polyps has been widely characterized, the specific events and signals that trigger this response are not well defined. [58]

Finally, pathogens can contribute directly and indirectly to the pathogenesis of CRS with polyps.

6.2.2 Extrinsic factors :

The responsibility of extrinsic factors in SFN does not seem to be accepted by the majority of authors, in particular the responsibility of a possible allergic factor. If not as factors that aggravate polyp pathology (see Favoring factors).

6.2.3 Intrinsic factors :

6.2.3.1 Histopathological factors :

This is evidenced by the active role of the nasal epithelium in cell proliferation, and by the rich inflammatory cell population found in polyps. The pathophysiology of PNS involves both epithelial and inflammatory factors.

A certain polymorphism seems to exist in the structure of polyps, although their histology is considered non-specific and has long been described as monomorphic.

While the fibro-edematous structure and inflammatory infiltrate remain the main histological features of polyps, other abnormalities are classically found: cellular atypia associated with patches of metaplasia; and areas of keratinization with flat metaplasia of columnar cells [100].

Classically, polyps can be classified histologically into edematous, glandular and fibrous polyps. This has led to the development of various theories concerning their formation, which no longer seem sufficient to explain the genesis of the disease.

Recent experimental work has given rise to the theory of "epithelial rupture" and abnormal repair of the respiratory mucosa [101].

The edematous polyp, by far the most common, was thought to be the result of increased vascular permeability, blocked lymphatic return and, more recently, disturbances in the ionic permeability of the nasal epithelium.

Multiple structural changes in capillaries are observed in polyps. Although the number of capillaries in the polyps appears to be significantly lower than in the mucosa of the lower turbinates, their permeability is much greater in the polyps. This could contribute to the formation of chorion edema. [102]

More recently, disorders of ionic permeability have been demonstrated in the epithelium of polyps, leading to increased sodium absorption and chlorine permeability, which may contribute to polyp formation. These chlorine permeability abnormalities appear to extend beyond the epithelium and reach the constituent fibroblasts of the polyp chorion, a role in fibroblast proliferation that still remains debated [103].

The glandular polyp, dominated by superficial glands with short excretory ducts and deep glands with long excretory ducts, obeys the theory of cystic dilatation of submucosal glands, known as the glandular theory. The size of polyps is proportional to the degree of dilatation of these glands. [104]

Ultimately, the fibrous type, in which fibroblastic proliferation and collagen fibers predominate, was considered a scarred or aged polyp. [105]

Based on this histological classification of polyps, various theories of their formation have been developed, but recent experimental work and a better understanding of the role of the nasal epithelium have challenged these theories. This histological classification now seems insufficient to explain the pathophysiological mechanisms of polyp formation.

6.2.3.2 Inflammatory cellular factors :

The common factor found in all SNPs is chronic inflammation of the respiratory mucosa, as evidenced by the rich cell population found in the polyps and surrounding nasal mucosa. The inflammatory infiltrate is made up of different cell types, depending on the nature of the polyposis.

- In so-called "primitive" polyposis, the most common, and those associated with the Fernand Widal triad, the inflammatory cellular infiltrate is characterized mainly by the presence of activated eosinophils.

- In so-called "secondary" polyposis, found in cystic fibrosis and ciliary dyskinesia, neutrophils predominate.

This subdivision is artificial and the richness in neutrophils seems to follow the local infection often present in so-called "secondary" polyposis, where defense processes are impaired [106].

6.2.3.2.1 Role of the eosinophilic polynuclear cell

Eosinophils are consistently found in "primitive" SFN, both in nasal secretions and within polyp tissue itself. They play an active role in perpetuating and sustaining the inflammatory reaction, thanks to their high content of membrane receptors and active mediators. This eosinophilic infiltration may be due to increased migration of circulating eosinophils towards the nasal mucosa, associated with exaggerated survival favoring their retention within this mucosa [9].

-Biological mechanisms of eosinophil recruitment: The recruitment of eosinophils to the site of inflammation is a complex process whose regulation depends on cytokines and chemokines. Interleukin (IL) 5 and *granulocyte-macrophage colony-stimulating factor* (GM-CSF) appear to play a key role in eosinophil recruitment [107,108].

The mechanisms of action of these two molecules are :

- induction of eosinophilic proliferation in bone marrow;

- the release of eosinophils from the bone marrow into the bloodstream;

- inhibition of eosinophil apoptosis.

Other molecules, including the chemokines eotaxin (EO) and *regulated on activation normal T cells expressed and secreted* (RANTES) , are significantly elevated in polyps. They are thought to play a role in the recruitment and activation of eosinophils. In addition, EO is thought to play a synergistic role with IL5 in activating eosinophil tissue migration. [109].

In addition to being secreted by inflammatory cells, including the eosinophil itself, these cytokines and chemokines are also secreted by respiratory epithelial cells present in the target inflammatory tissue.

-Biological mechanisms of eosinophil survival and tissue maintenance: The maintenance of eosinophilic infiltration in SFN is explained by :

- inhibition of eosinophil apoptosis;

- the action of adhesion molecules expressed in target tissues.

The *intercellular adhesion molecule-1* (ICAM-1) is highly expressed on the surface of activated respiratory epithelial cells within polyps, and is the main carrier of eosinophil attachment. ICAM-1 is expressed under the influence of pro-inflammatory mediators released by mast cells, eosinophils and the epithelial cells themselves.

As in the case of eosinophil recruitment, there is a real loop stimulating the survival and maintenance of eosinophils within the polyps themselves [110,111].

-Mechanisms initiating tissue eosinophilia in polyposis: Several mechanisms initiating tissue eosinophilia in polyposis have been proposed.

_ **The role of IgE-dependent allergy** : The role of allergy in polyposis remains debated, but the majority agree that although it is an attractive mechanism to explain tissue eosinophilia in polyposis, it cannot be considered a univocal cause of polyposis.

Thus, while IgE-dependent allergy alone cannot explain the development of SFN, it seems legitimate to think that it may contribute to the tissue eosinophilia of polyposis, when these two conditions are associated. [112,113]

_ **The role of local infection:** Bacterial or viral infections have long been considered opportunistic in SNP, most often secondary to retention after nasal obstruction.

Nonetheless, three mechanisms linked to local nasosinus infection have been suggested in an attempt to explain eosinophilia in SFN:

- the first mechanism is that of a bacterial allergy developed following a local infection, responsible for chronic eosinophilic inflammation of the nasal mucosa [70] ;

- the second mechanism is the development of a chronic inflammatory reaction, following local rhinovirus infection, which induces specific IL8 production by nasal epithelial cells. This IL8 is involved in neutrophil recruitment, leading to the establishment of a secondary inflammatory reaction. On-site persistence of neutrophils could lead to chronic inflammation and recruitment of other inflammatory cells. Eosinophilic infiltration is therefore secondary to neutrophilic infiltration, and could under certain conditions lead to the development of polyposis [69,114,115] ;

- the third mechanism is local stress on the nasal mucosa. This would be induced by an infection responsible for an influx of eosinophils secondary to the local expression of kinins, leading to the establishment of a local tissue inflammatory reaction. This neurogenic inflammation, combined with nasal hyperadrenergy, leads to tissue eosinophilic infiltration, characteristic of *non allergic rhinitis eosinophil syndrome* (NARES), which is known to have the potential to develop into polyposis. [116,117].

Role of leukotrienes: their role in SFN has been suggested on the basis of the pathophysiological mechanisms encountered in aspirin intolerance. This involves a disturbance in the degradation metabolism of membrane phospholipids, particularly arachidonic acid, resulting in exaggerated production of leukotrienes, with a significant reduction in the ratio of cyclooxygenase degradation products (thromboxane B2, prostaglandins E2 and F1 alpha) to lipo-oxygenase degradation products (leukotrienes B4 and C4). 117,118][

The latter, with their pro-inflammatory and vasoactive properties, provoke a chronic inflammatory reaction with tissue eosinophilia. This eosinophilia is formed by the combined action of secondarily released pro-inflammatory molecules and leukotriene B4, which has a chemotactic effect on eosinophils. The recruited and activated eosinophils are able to participate in the self-perpetuation of the inflammatory reaction by secreting various cytokines, C4 leukotrienes and prostaglandins. [9,119]

Role of the tissue microenvironment: epithelial, endothelial and fibroblast cells play a predominant role in the generation and maintenance of the inflammatory response. This group of cells, self-activated by the expression of pro-inflammatory factors, participates in the recruitment and maintenance of eosinophilia in the target tissue. This self-activation of the various cell groups making up polyps provides the basis for the microenvironmental theory. [9]

The role of an autocrine eosinophil activation disorder: This is based on a primary disorder of eosinophil physiology, which would lead to their auto-activation, ensuring their survival and maintenance in the target tissue. The primary abnormality could lie in the eosinophil membrane receptor for IL5, and would involve this cytokine predominantly in the "autocrine" theory of tissue eosinophilia in SNP. [107]

6.2.3.2.2 Role of mast cells :

The role of mast cells in SFN is controversial. The discovery of mast cell growth factors, including the *stem cell factor* (SCF) within the polyp, supports the hypothesis of mast cell recruitment and activation, participating in eosinophilic activation via pro-inflammatory cytokines secreted by mast cells. This hypothesis is supported by other studies showing mast cell infiltration in polyposis, independently of any associated allergy. [120,121]

6.2.3.2.3 Role of lymphocytes :

The role of lymphocytes in SFN is also debated. Some authors had put forward a cell-mediated dysimmune hypothesis with secondary eosinophilic infiltration, following the demonstration of a significant decrease in the ratio of TH8 so-called suppressor lymphocytes to TH 4 so-called helper lymphocytes in SFN.

In the end, further work failed to confirm this hypothesis, by showing comparable TH8/TH4 ratios between polyps and surrounding tissues. This suggests that lymphocytes in polyposis are a feature of the inflammatory reaction, and not of polyposis itself. 9,122,123][

6.2.3.2.4 Role of neutrophils :

Polynuclear neutrophils may play an active role in so-called "secondary" polyposis, given the frequency of superinfections in these areas.

6.2.3.3 Epithelial cellular factors: the role of the epithelium

The epithelium of the respiratory tract is constantly subjected to a variety of external stresses, which can damage epithelial cells, detach them from the basement membrane, or even rupture the basement membrane. In any case, restoring the structural and functional integrity of the epithelium requires a repair process combining migration, proliferation and differentiation of respiratory epithelial cells. These phenomena are closely dependent on interactions between the cells themselves and between the cells and the extracellular matrix. [124]

Direct involvement of epithelial cells in the mechanism of chronic inflammation: The subdivision into primary eosinophilic polyposis and secondary polyposis without eosinophils enables a separate and more precise study of the pathophysiological mechanisms of SFN.

- Eosinophilic or primary polyposis :

During the inflammatory reaction, the nasal epithelium plays an active role, thanks to various mediators that both recruit and activate inflammatory cells, which in turn secrete pro-inflammatory mediators. These molecules participate in the recruitment and activation of other inflammatory cells, while acting on the epithelial and structural cells (fibroblasts and endothelial cells) of the respiratory mucosa.

The epithelial cell is thus a key player in the inflammatory reaction, especially as it is in the front line when faced with stimuli and aggression from the external environment.

Inflammatory mediators, including cytokines, play a central role through their powerful pro-inflammatory and, in some cases, anti-inflammatory actions, as well as through their network organization.

Schematically, during the inflammatory reaction, a distinction is made between cytokines of the early response and cytokines of the late response:

- the "early" cytokines of the initiation and propagation phases of inflammation are characterized by their powerful but unspecific actions *(tumor necrosis factor* [TNF-a] and IL1).

- late" cytokines, known as amplification-phase cytokines, are characterized by their more targeted actions on particular cell types (interferons [IFN], *colony stimulating factor* [CSF], *transforming growth factor* [TGF] , chemokines, IL3, IL4, IL5, IL6).

Eosinophils are known to be the key inflammatory cells in primary polyposis. Most work has focused on characterizing the expression of the cytokines most specific to the recruitment and activation of this cell: IL3, IL5, IL8; GM-CSF and RANTES. [125[125-127]

The epithelium may also play a role in the inflammatory process of polyps, through the secretion of mediators other than cytokines. Epithelial cells secrete arachidonic acid derivatives with powerful pro-inflammatory properties, such as leukotrienes and prostaglandins. Add to this the nasal and sinus epithelial cells, which express the constitutive form of NO synthetase (enzyme enabling synthesis of nitric oxide) and are an important source of NO, which is a mediator with varied actions and notably involved in inflammation. [128]

The overexpression by epithelial cells of surface proteins from major histocompatibility complex type II (HLA-DR) , as well as cell adhesion proteins (ICAM-1) , which attract inflammatory cells locally, appear to participate in the local action and confer immunological competence. [9]

All in all, epithelial cells play an important role in the complex network of cellular and molecular factors involved in the chronic nasal inflammation that characterizes eosinophilic polyposis. [112,129]

- Non-eosinophilic" or secondary polyposis

The inflammatory mechanisms involved in "eosinophil-free" polyposis appear to be different, and are probably specific to underlying conditions such as cystic fibrosis or congenital ciliary dyskinesia.

These pathologies represent special cases of chronic nasal inflammation linked to a congenital defect in epithelial cells, which are central to the inflammatory reaction and thus to the pathophysiology of SFN. [9]

_ **Direct involvement of epithelial cells in polyp development:**

The mechanisms of nasosinus polyp formation and growth are still open to debate.

Initially, polyp formation was considered to be an edematous herniation of the mucosa associated with cystic dilatation of the submucosal glands. 105,130][

The recent hypothesis is based on the notion of a primitive break in the continuity of the epithelium and basement membrane. Thus, connective tissue containing macrophages, fibroblasts and inflammatory cells infiltrates through this break, and the epithelium then progresses from the edges of the defect in both directions:

- on the one hand, it lines the conjunctival hernia;

- on the other hand, it sinks into the lamina propria and forms microcavities.

These microcavities enlarge and fuse, at the same time as their epithelium differentiates with the appearance of ciliated and secretory cells. As they fuse, these cavities cleave the epithelium, resulting in the individualization of a polyp **(Figure 23)**. [9]

In view of the experimental work carried out on animals and the changes observed in situ in the polyps, the development of nasosinusal polyps could be considered as an "exaggerated" phenomenon of tissue repair. This mechanism involves :

- inflammatory cells ;

- mesenchymal and endothelial cells ;

- but above all epithelial cells.

The dysregulation of the repair process is complex. Schematically, various growth factors are inappropriately secreted by inflammatory, epithelial and mesenchymal cells in the nasal mucosa, leading to polyp formation. As inflammation and epithelial repair are intimately linked, this process of exaggerated repair could be incorporated into the concept of microenvironmental theory, which conceptualizes runaway inflammation in the nasal mucosa. Thus, chronic inflammation and polyp development would be two interdependent pathophysiological mechanisms in which epithelial cells play a major role. [9,10,124]

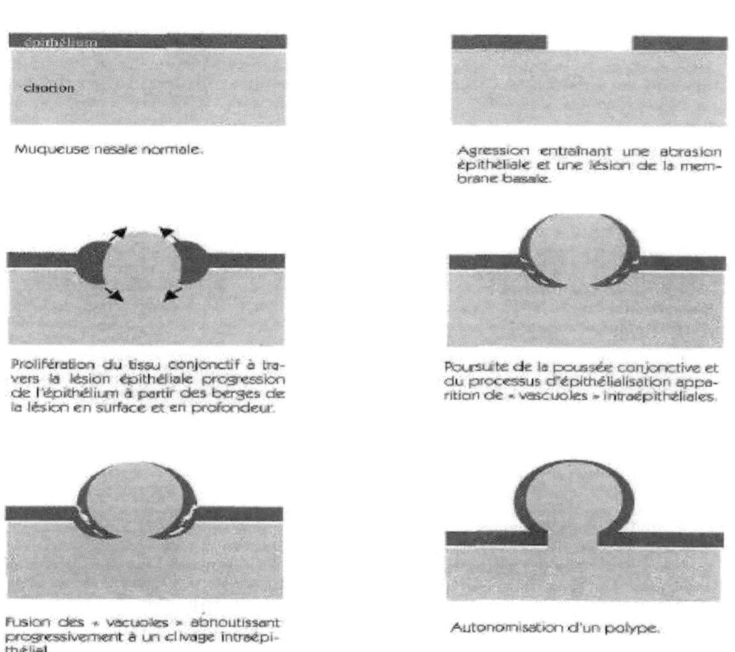

Figure 23*Schematic representation of the stages in the development of a nasosinus polyp in an experimental animal model after Norlander et al.*
[9]

6.2.4 The evo-devo theory of nose formation:

This theory conceives of the human and mammalian nasal organ in general as an evolutionary assembly of three different noses that repeat during development, and nasal polyposis as a specific disease of the olfactory nose. [30]

The olfactory nose developed in the first vertebrates, which were fish, by invagination of the ectodermal olfactory placodes above the oral cavity towards the primitive brain, establishing a connection between the chemosensory cells of the olfactory placodes and the primitive neural tissue via a mesenchyme that gave rise to the prechordal cartilages, the undisputed phylogenetic precursors of the human ethmoid bone.

Bipedalism is probably at the origin of the human compartmentalization of the ethmoid into olfactory clefts, of which only the superior recess shelters the olfactory mucosa, and into lateral masses of which the original olfactory mucosa may have regressed into a vestigial olfactory mucosa. [131]

The respiratory nose developed secondarily at the expense of the oral cavity, underneath the olfactory nose, by remodeling and repositioning the secondary palate bones of the first terrestrial tetrapods, progressively displacing the respiratory orifices of the amphibian olfactory nose (called primary choanae, of which the incisive canal represents the vestigial state in humans), which open behind the primary palate, towards the rear during the evolution of therapsids, the ancestors of mammals. Between the oral cavity and the olfactory nose, there are two respiratory corridors that open at the glottis via secondary choanae. The floor of the olfactory nose that separates it anatomically from the respiratory nose, called the transverse blade in mammals, has disappeared in man, probably as a result of the acquisition of bipedalism. No aquatic animal has paranasal sinuses. In humans, the paranasal sinuses only begin to develop after birth. [131,132]

In the evo-devo conception, nasal polyposis is a chronic inflammatory disease of the vestigial olfactory mucosa of the ethmoid.

If the mucosa of the lateral masses of the human ethmoid really is the result of a degeneration of the olfactory mucosa that originally lined the ethmo-turbinals, as a result of their curved, onion-bulb-like stacking during evolution and development. It would then be possible that this involution of the olfactory mucosa is not complete or perfect in all individuals, leaving some elements of the original olfactory mucosa, such as Jourdan cells or simply self-antigens, to persist in some. [30,31,133]

6.2.5 Aspirin intolerance:

The originator of the Widal triad, aspirin has been widely used for its antipyretic, analgesic and anti-inflammatory properties since its discovery in 1899. It has numerous side effects, including rashes, asthma and angioedema. The first case of aspirin intolerance was described by Hirschberg in 1902, concerning urticaria and angioedema (Quincke's edema) with nasal obstruction following aspirin intake. [134]

Initially, intolerance was considered rare and related solely to aspirin, until it was extended to all NSAIDs and other substances such as analgesics and certain drug or food additives, following the publications of Samter [78]Settipane [76]Slavin [135] and Szczeklik [136]. [137]

The allergic theory was long implicated in the phenomenon of aspirin intolerance, but has now been abandoned in favor of a biochemical mechanism involving cyclooxygenase (COX). [137[137-139]

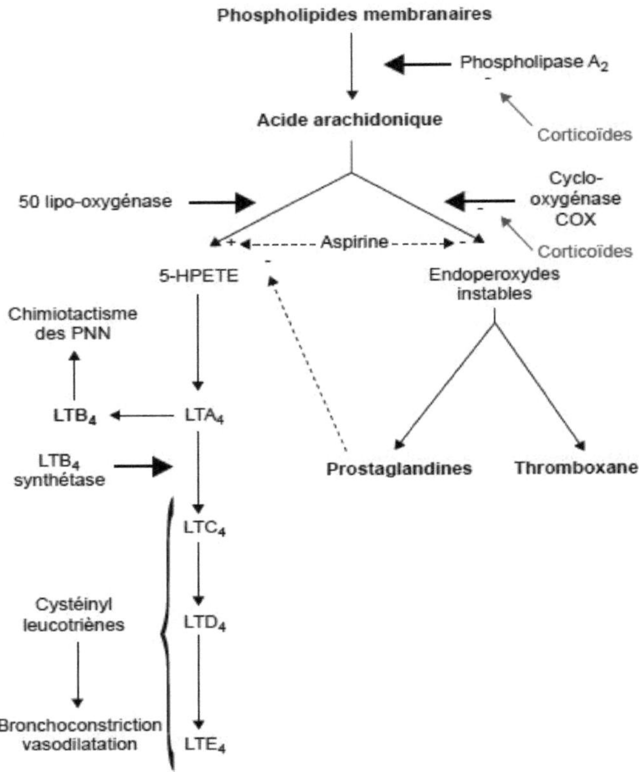

Figure 24*Degradation of membrane phospholipids and action of corticoids (after Monneret-Vautrin).* [140]

(LT: leukotriene; PNN: neutrophils; 5-HPETE: 5-hydroperoxyeicosatetraenoic acid).

Aspirin intolerance can be divided into three categories [136] :

- type A (15% of cases): respiratory symptoms (asthma and rhinitis);

- type B (75% of cases): combining urticaria and angioedema;

- type C (10% of cases): special clinical forms such as erythema, exanthema, Stevens-Johnson syndrome or Lyell syndrome.

Symptoms may be cutaneous and/or respiratory, occurring on average an hour and a half after ingestion of a dose of 10 to 100 mg aspirin.

In the current theory, which accords a predominant role to COX types 1 and 2, NSAIDs inhibit COX , resulting in an imbalance in arachidonic acid metabolism in favour of one of the accessory pathways, responsible for a (**Figure 24**) [141[141-144] :

- inhibition of prostaglandin synthesis ;

- hyperactivity of 5-lipo-oxygenase responsible for excessive production of leukotrienes (LTC4 , LTD4 and LTE4), mediators known for their powerful inflammatory action;

- increased expression of LTC4 synthetase.

This accumulation of leukotrienes is responsible for the clinical symptoms observed.

6.2.6 Fungal allergy :

Fungal sinusitis was first described in 1976 by Safirstein, who admitted the existence of forms associating polyposis and intrasinusal mycotic infections. [145]

It was not until the 1980s that the concept of allergic fungal sinusitis or Katzenstein syndrome was born. [146-148]

Many uncertainties persist concerning the pathophysiology of this disease. For most authors, it is linked to a hypersensitivity reaction to the initial fungal element, with a combination of type I (IgE) and III (immune complexes) immunological reactions according to the Gell and Coombs classification.

The disease begins with the inhalation and trapping *of* fungal spores by sinus mucus. The release of antigenic material stimulates the production of IgE, IgG and IgA. As a result, aspergillary antigens react with IgE-sensitized mast cells. The antigen-antibody reaction then induces mast cell degranulation, with the release of inflammatory mediators.

These allergic reactions lead to edema and inflammation, resulting in ostial obstructions and intra-sinus stasis.

This is a favorable environment for fungal proliferation, which in turn increases the quantity of antigens, generating what is known as a vicious circle leading to the formation of mucin. [9,141,149]

Since the pathophysiology of the disease remains unclear, Marple proposes a pathophysiological scheme involving various parameters (**Figure 25**). [150]

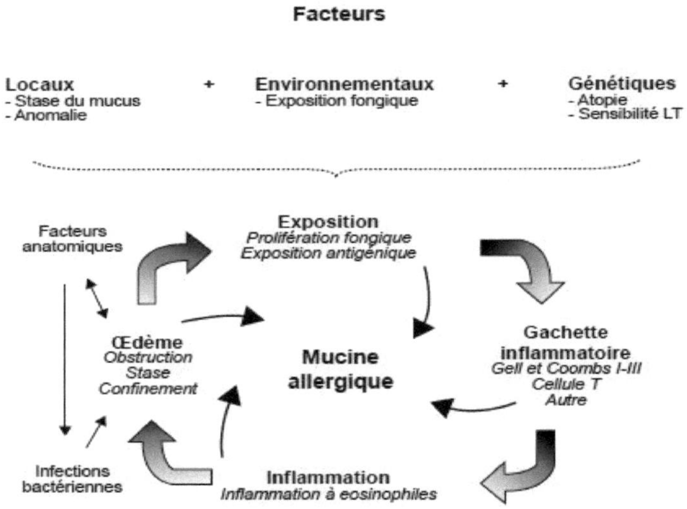

Figure 25*Pathophysiology of allergic fungal sinusitis formation (after Marple).* [140]

References :

[2] " European Position Paper on Rhinosinusitis and Nasal Polyps 2012. - PubMed - NCBI." https://www.ncbi.nlm.nih.gov/pubmed/22764607 (accessed May 16, 2019).

[9] Peynegre, Freche, Fontanel, *la polypose naso sinusienne*. Société Française d'Oto-rhino-laryngologie et de Chirurgie de la Face et du Cou, 2000.

[10] T. M. Önerci and B. J. Ferguson, eds, *Nasal Polyposis: Pathogenesis, Medical and Surgical Treatment*. Berlin Heidelberg: Springer-Verlag, 2010.

[30] R. Jankowski, *The Evo-Devo Origin of the Nose, Anterior Skull Base and Midface*. Paris: Springer-Verlag, 2013.

[31] R. Jankowski, C. Perrot, D. T. Nguyen, and C. Rumeau, "Structure of the lateral masses of the ethmoid by curved stacking of the endoturbinals", *Ann. Fr. Oto-Rhino-Laryngol. Pathol. Cervico-Faciale*, vol. 133, n° 5, pp. 293-298, Nov. 2016, doi: 10.1016/j.aforl.2016.02.010.

[57] K. Larsen and M. Tos, "The estimated incidence of symptomatic nasal polyps", *Acta Otolaryngol. (Stockh.)*, vol. 122, n° 2, pp. 179-182, March 2002.

[58] W. W. Stevens, R. P. Schleimer, and R. C. Kern, "Chronic Rhinosinusitis with Nasal Polyps," *J. Allergy Clin. Immunol. Pract.* vol. 4, n° 4, pp. 565-572, Jul. 2016, doi: 10.1016/j.jaip.2016.04.012.

[59] Falliers CJ, "Familial coincidence of asthma, aspirin intolerance and nasal polyposis," *Ann Allergy*, n° 32, pp. 65-69, 1974.

[60] Havas TE, Motbey JA, Gullane PJ, "Prevalence of incidental abnormalities on computed tomographic scans of the paranasal sinuses," *Arch Otolaryngol Head Neck Surg*, n° 114, pp. 856-859, 1988.

[61] Suttner HJ, Hosemann W, Rockelein G, "Histologische Stufenschnitt-Untersuchungen an Siebbeinpräparaten bei Polyposis nasi.", *Eur Arch Otorhinolaryngol*, n° 249, p. 360, 1992.

[62] G. A. Settipane, "Epidemiology of nasal polyps", *Allergy Asthma Proc.* vol. 17, n° 5, pp. 231-236, Oct. 1996.

[63] G. A. Settipane and F. H. Chafee, "Nasal polyps in asthma and rhinitis. A review of 6,037 patients," *J. Allergy Clin. Immunol*, vol. 59, n° 1, pp. 17-21, Jan. 1977.

[64] Crampette L, Serrano E, Klossek JM, Rugina M, Rouvier P, and Peynegre R et al, "Etude épidémiologique prospective multicentrique française (Groupe ORLI) de la pathologie pneumo-allergologique associée à la polypose naso-sinusienne.", 2001. http://www.revue-laryngologie.com/detail.lasso?id=cbfc13e988b38c05 (accessed May 18, 2019).

[65] N. Mygind, "Nasal polyposis, eosinophil dominated inflammation, and allergy", *Thorax*, vol. 55, n° 90002, pp. 79S - 83, Oct. 2000, doi: 10.1136/thorax.55.suppl_2.S79.

[66] Jacobs RL, Freda AJ, Culver WG, "Primary nasal polyposis," *Ann Allergy*, n° 51, pp. 500-505, 1983.

[67] P. K. Keith *et al*, "Nasal polyps: effects of seasonal allergen exposure", *J. Allergy Clin. Immunol*, vol. 93, n° 3, pp. 567-574, March 1994.

[68] J. E. Waxman, J. G. Spector, S. R. Sale, and A. L. Katzenstein, "Allergic Aspergillus sinusitis: concepts in diagnosis and treatment of a new clinical entity", *The Laryngoscope*, vol. 97, n° 3 Pt 1, pp. 261-266, March 1987.

[69] J. Allen, R. Eisma, G. Leonard, D. Lafreniere, and D. Kreutzer, "Interleukin-8 expression in human nasal polyps," *Otolaryngol. Head Neck Surg.* vol. 117, n° 5, pp. 535-541, Nov. 1997, doi: 10.1016/S0194-5998(97)70027-5.

[70] E. Calenoff, J. T. McMahan, G. D. Herzon, R. C. Kern, G. D. Ghadge, and D. G. Hanson, "Bacterial allergy in nasal polyposis. A new method for quantifying specific IgE", *Arch. Otolaryngol. Head Neck Surg.* vol. 119, n° 8, pp. 830-836, August 1993.

[71] Noah TL, Henderson FW, Wortman IA, Devlin RB, Handy J, Koren HS et al, "Nasal cytokine production in viral acute upper respiratory infection of childhood," n° 171, pp. 584-592, 1995.

[72] C. Grigoreas, D. Vourdas, K. Petalas, G. Simeonidis, I. Demeroutis, and T. Tsioulos, "Nasal polyps in patients with rhinitis and asthma," *Allergy Asthma Proc.* vol. 23, n° 3, pp. 169-174, June 2002.

[73] S. Robinson, R. Douglas, and P.-J. Wormald, "The relationship between atopy and chronic rhinosinusitis," *Am. J. Rhinol.* vol. 20, n° 6, pp. 625-628, Dec. 2006.

[74] A. N. Pearlman *et al*, "Relationships between severity of chronic rhinosinusitis and nasal polyposis, asthma, and atopy," *Am. J. Rhinol. Allergy*, vol. 23, n° 2, pp. 145-148, Apr. 2009, doi: 10.2500/ajra.2009.23.3284.

[75] W. A. Greisner and G. A. Settipane, "Hereditary Factor for Nasal Polyps," *Allergy Asthma Proc.* vol. 17, n° 5, pp. 283-286, Sept. 1996, doi: 10.2500/108854196778662192.

[76] G. A. Settipane, "Aspirin sensitivity and allergy," *Biomed. Pharmacother. Biomedecine Pharmacother.* vol. 42, n° 8, pp. 493-498, 1988.

[77] N. A. Cohen, J. S. Widelitz, A. G. Chiu, J. N. Palmer, and D. W. Kennedy, "Familial aggregation of sinonasal polyps correlates with severity of disease," *Otolaryngol.--Head Neck Surg. Off. J. Am. Acad. Otolaryngol.-Head Neck Surg.* vol. 134, n° 4, pp. 601-604, Apr. 2006, doi: 10.1016/j.otohns.2005.11.042.

[78] M. Samter and R. F. Beers, "Intolerance to aspirin. Clinical studies and consideration of its pathogenesis," *Ann. Intern. Med*, vol. 68, n° 5, pp. 975-983, May 1968.

[79] W. W. Pleskow, D. D. Stevenson, D. A. Mathison, R. A. Simon, M. Schatz, and R. S. Zeiger, "Aspirin-sensitive rhinosinusitis/asthma:

spectrum of adverse reactions to aspirin," *J. Allergy Clin. Immunol*, vol. 71, n° 6, pp. 574-579, June 1983.
[80] J.-E. Kim and S. E. Kountakis, "The prevalence of Samter's triad in patients undergoing functional endoscopic sinus surgery," *Ear. Nose. Throat J.*, vol. 86, n° 7, pp. 396-399, July 2007.
[81] L. Probst, P. Stoney, E. Jeney, and M. Hawke, "Nasal polyps, bronchial asthma and aspirin sensitivity," *J. Otolaryngol.* vol. 21, n° 1, pp. 60-65, Feb. 1992.

[82] D. A. Moneret-Vautrin, V. Hsieh, M. Wayoff, J. L. Guyot, C. Mouton, and Y. Maria, "Nonallergic rhinitis with eosinophilia syndrome a precursor of the triad: nasal polyposis, intrinsic asthma, and intolerance to aspirin," *Ann. Allergy*, vol. 64, n° 6, pp. 513-518, June 1990.
[83] M. L. Kowalski *et al*, "Differential metabolism of arachidonic acid in nasal polyp epithelial cells cultured from aspirin-sensitive and aspirin-tolerant patients," *Am. J. Respir. Crit. Care Med.* vol. 161, n° 2 Pt 1, pp. 391-398, Feb 2000, doi: 10.1164/ajrccm.161.2.9902034.
[84] P. S. Batra *et al*, "Outcome analysis of endoscopic sinus surgery in patients with nasal polyps and asthma", *The Laryngoscope*, vol. 113, n° 10, pp. 1703-1706, Oct. 2003.
[85] D. Glass and R. G. Amedee, "Allergic Fungal Rhinosinusitis: A Review," *Ochsner J.*, vol. 11, n° 3, pp. 271-275, 2011.
[86] J. P. Bent and F. A. Kuhn, "Diagnosis of allergic fungal sinusitis," *Otolaryngol.--Head Neck Surg. Off. J. Am. Acad. Otolaryngol.-Head Neck Surg.* vol. 111, n° 5, pp. 580-588, Nov. 1994, doi: 10.1177/019459989411100508.
[87] S. B. Kupferberg, J. P. Bent, and F. A. Kuhn, "Prognosis for allergic fungal sinusitis," *Otolaryngol.--Head Neck Surg. Off. J. Am. Acad. Otolaryngol.-Head Neck Surg.* vol. 117, n° 1, pp. 35-41, July 1997, doi: 10.1016/S0194-59989770203-1.
[88] J. P. Corey, "Allergic fungal sinusitis," *Otolaryngol. Clin. North Am.* vol. 25, n° 1, pp. 225-230, Feb. 1992.
[89] S. C. Manning and M. Holman, "Further evidence for allergic pathophysiology in allergic fungal sinusitis", *The Laryngoscope*, vol. 108, n° 10, pp. 1485-1496, Oct. 1998.
[90] S. K. Wise, M. D. Ghegan, E. Gorham, and R. J. Schlosser, "Socioeconomic factors in the diagnosis of allergic fungal rhinosinusitis," *Otolaryngol.--Head Neck Surg. Off. J. Am. Acad. Otolaryngol.-Head Neck Surg.* vol. 138, n° 1, p. 38-42, Jan. 2008, doi: 10.1016/j.otohns.2007.10.020.
[91] C. Bachert, P. Gevaert, P. Howarth, G. Holtappels, P. van Cauwenberge, and S. G. O. Johansson, "IgE to Staphylococcus

aureus enterotoxins in serum is related to severity of asthma," *J. Allergy Clin. Immunol.* vol. 111, n° 5, pp. 1131-1132, May 2003.

[92] T. Van Zele *et al*, "Differentiation of chronic sinus diseases by measurement of inflammatory mediators", *Allergy*, vol. 61, n° 11, pp. 1280-1289, Nov. 2006, doi: 10.1111/j.1398-9995.2006.01225.x.

[93] " Transforming growth factor beta abrogates the effects of hematopoietins on eosinophils and induces their apoptosis," *J. Exp. Med.* vol. 179, n° 3, pp. 1041-1045, March 1994.

[94] SYUHADA O1, SHALINI P1, LIM WK1, AMMAR A1, SURIA HAYATI MP2, ANEEZA KHAIRIYAH WH1, GENDEH BS1, NORAIDAH M2, SALINA H1, "Malaysian Nasal Polyps: Eosinophil or Neutrophil-Predominant," *Med & Health*, n° 11(1), pp. 56-61, 2016.

[95] N. Zhang, G. Holtappels, C. Claeys, G. Huang, P. van Cauwenberge, and C. Bachert, "Pattern of inflammation and impact of Staphylococcus aureus enterotoxins in nasal polyps from southern China", *Am. J. Rhinol.* vol. 20, n° 4, p. 445-450, August 2006.

[96] J.-W. Kim, S.-L. Hong, Y.-K. Kim, C. H. Lee, Y.-G. Min, and C.-S. Rhee, "Histological and immunological features of non-eosinophilic nasal polyps," *Otolaryngol.--Head Neck Surg. Off. J. Am. Acad. Otolaryngol.-Head Neck Surg.* vol. 137, n° 6, pp. 925-930, Dec. 2007, doi: 10.1016/j.otohns.2007.07.036.

[97] C. Ozcan, H. Zeren, D. U. Talas, M. Küçükoğlu, and K. Görür, "Antrochoanal polyp: a transmission electron and light microscopic study", *Eur. Arch. Oto-Rhino-Laryngol. Off. J. Eur. Fed. Oto-Rhino-Laryngol. Soc. EUFOS Affil. Ger. Soc. Oto-Rhino-Laryngol. - Head Neck Surg.* vol. 262, n° 1, p. 55-60, Jan. 2005, doi: 10.1007/s00405-003-0729-1.

[98] M. B. Soyka *et al*, "Defective epithelial barrier in chronic rhinosinusitis: The regulation of tight junctions by IFN-γ and IL-4", *J. Allergy Clin. Immunol.* vol. 130, n° 5, pp. 1087-1096.e10, Nov. 2012, doi: 10.1016/j.jaci.2012.05.052.

[99] K. L. Pothoven *et al*, "Oncostatin M promotes mucosal epithelial barrier dysfunction, and its expression is increased in patients with eosinophilic mucosal disease," *J. Allergy Clin. Immunol.* vol. 136, n° 3, pp. 737-746.e4, Sept. 2015, doi: 10.1016/j.jaci.2015.01.043.

[100] A. R. Baird, O. Hilmi, P. S. White, and A. J. Robertson, "Epithelial atypia and squamous metaplasia in nasal polyps," *J. Laryngol. Otol.* vol. 112, n° 8, pp. 755-757, August 1998.

[101] C. Freche, J. P. Fontanel, and R. Peynegre, *Nasosinus polyposis*. 2000.

[102]K. Watanabe and A. Komatsuzaki, "Ultrastructural findings of capillaries in nasal polyps", *Rhinology*, vol. 30, n° 1, pp. 49-56, March 1992.
[103]J. M. Bernstein, J. Gorfien, B. Noble, and J. R. Yankaskas, "Nasal polyposis: immunohistochemistry and bioelectrical findings (a hypothesis for the development of nasal polyps)," *J. Allergy Clin. Immunol*, vol. 99, n° 2, pp. 165-175, Feb. 1997.
[104]H. Kakoi and F. Hiraide, "A histological study of formation and growth of nasal polyps", *Acta Otolaryngol. (Stockh.)*, vol. 103, n° 1-2, pp. 137-144, Feb. 1987.
[105]Z. Krajina and A. Zirdum, "Histochemical analysis of nasal polyps", *Acta Otolaryngol. (Stockh.)*, vol. 103, n° 5-6, pp. 435-440, June 1987.
[106]J. M. Rowe-Jones, N. Trendell-Smith, M. Shembekar, and I. S. Mackay, "Polypoid rhinosinusitis in patients with host defense deficiencies: cellular infiltration and disease severity", *Rhinology*, vol. 35, n° 3, pp. 113-117, Sept. 1997.
[107]M. Kramer and G. Rasp, "Nasal polyposis: eosinophils and interleukin-5", *Allergy*, vol. 54, n° 7, pp. 669-680, Dec. 2001, doi: 10.1034/j.1398-9995.1999.00095.x.
[108]" Nasal interleukin-5, immunoglobulin E, eosinophilic cationic protein, and soluble intercellular adhesion molecule-1 in chronic sinusitis, allergic ... - PubMed - NCBI". https://www.ncbi.nlm.nih.gov/pubmed/10852530 (accessed May 21, 2019).
[109]J. S. Allen, R. Eisma, D. LaFreniere, G. Leonard, and D. Kreutzer, "Characterization of the eosinophil chemokine RANTES in nasal polyps," *Ann. Otol. Rhinol. Laryngol.* vol. 107, n° 5 Pt 1, pp. 416-420, May 1998, doi: 10.1177/000348949810700510.
[110]M. B. Resnick and P. F. Weller, "Mechanisms of eosinophil recruitment," *Am. J. Respir. Cell Mol. Biol.* vol. 8, n° 4, pp. 349-355, Apr. 1993, doi: 10.1165/ajrcmb/8.4.349.
[111]D. Adamko, P. Lacy, and R. Moqbel, "Mechanisms of eosinophil recruitment and activation," *Curr. Allergy Asthma Rep.* vol. 2, n° 2, pp. 107-116, March 2002.
[112]J. M. Bernstein, J. Gorfien, and B. Noble, "Role of allergy in nasal polyposis: a review," *Otolaryngol.--Head Neck Surg. Off. J. Am. Acad. Otolaryngol.-Head Neck Surg.* vol. 113, n° 6, pp. 724-732, Dec. 1995, doi: 10.1016/S0194-59989570012-9.
[113]R. Jankowski, "Eosinophils in the pathophysiology of nasal polyposis," *Acta Otolaryngol. (Stockh.)*, vol. 116, n° 2, pp. 160-163, March 1996.

[114]T. L. Noah *et al*, "Nasal cytokine production in viral acute upper respiratory infection of childhood," *J. Infect. Dis.* vol. 171, n° 3, pp. 584-592, March 1995, doi: 10.1093/infdis/171.3.584.

[115]M. C. Subauste, D. B. Jacoby, S. M. Richards, and D. Proud, "Infection of a human respiratory epithelial cell line with rhinovirus. Induction of cytokine release and modulation of susceptibility to infection by cytokine exposure," *J. Clin. Invest.* vol. 96, n° 1, pp. 549-557, July 1995, doi: 10.1172/JCI118067.

[116]D. J. Dusser, D. B. Jacoby, T. D. Djokic, I. Rubinstein, D. B. Borson, and J. A. Nadel, "Virus induces airway hyperresponsiveness to tachykinins: role of neutral endopeptidase," *J. Appl. Physiol. Bethesda Md 1985*, vol. 67, n° 4, pp. 1504-1511, Oct. 1989, doi: 10.1152/jappl.1989.67.4.1504.

[117]D. Moneret-Vautrin, Wayoff M, V. Hsieh, Y. Maria, and R. Jankowski, "Le NARES, maillon évolutif de la triade de Widal," *Ann Otolaryngol*, n° 106, pp. 47-50, 1989.

[118]S. Pinto *et al*, "Cyclooxygenase and lipoxygenase metabolite generation in nasal polyps," *Prostaglandins Leukot. Essent. Fatty Acids*, vol. 57, n° 6, pp. 533-537, Dec. 1997.

[119]P. Demoly, L. Crampette, B. Lebel, A. M. Campbell, M. Mondain, and J. Bousquet, "Expression of cyclo-oxygenase 1 and 2 proteins in upper respiratory mucosa," *Clin. Exp. Allergy J. Br. Soc. Allergy Clin. Immunol.* vol. 28, n° 3, pp. 278-283, March 1998.

[120]R. Pawliczak, M. L. Kowalski, M. Danilewicz, M. Wagrowska-Danilewicz, and A. Lewandowski, "Distribution of Mast Cells and Eosinophils in Nasal Polyps from Atopic and Nonatopic Subjects: A Morphometric Study," *Am. J. Rhinol.* vol. 11, n° 4, pp. 257-262, July 1997, doi: 10.2500/105065897781446711.

[121]Y. K. Kim, N. Nakagawa, K. Nakano, I. Sulakvelidze, J. Dolovich, and J. Denburg, "Stem cell factor in nasal polyposis and allergic rhinitis: increased expression by structural cells is suppressed by in vivo topical corticosteroids," *J. Allergy Clin. Immunol*, vol. 100, n° 3, p. 389-399, Sept. 1997.

[122]A. E. Stoop, H. A. van der Heijden, J. Biewenga, and S. van der Baan, "Lymphocytes and nonlymphoid cells in human nasal polyps," *J. Allergy Clin. Immunol*, vol. 87, n° 2, pp. 470-475, Feb. 1991.

[123]A. Linder, A. Karlsson-Parra, C. Hirvelä, L. Jonsson, A. Köling, and O. Sjöberg, "Immunocompetent cells in human nasal polyps and normal mucosa", *Rhinology*, vol. 31, n° 3, pp. 125-129, Sept. 1993.

[124]C. G. Persson, J. S. Erjefält, I. Erjefält, M. C. Korsgren, M. C. Nilsson, and F. Sundler, "Epithelial shedding--restitution as a causative process in airway inflammation," *Clin. Exp. Allergy J. Br. Soc. Allergy Clin. Immunol.* vol. 26, n° 7, pp. 746-755, July 1996.

[125] A. J. Polito and D. Proud, "Epithelia cells as regulators of airway inflammation," *J. Allergy Clin. Immunol.* vol. 102, n° 5, pp. 714-718, Nov. 1998.
[126] J. Kelley, "Cytokines of the lung," *Am. Rev. Respir. Dis.* vol. 141, n° 3, pp. 765-788, March 1990, doi: 10.1164/ajrccm/141.3.765.
[127] Cavaillon J, Haeffner-Cavaillon N, "cytokines et inflammation", *Rev Prat*, n° 43, p. 547-552, 1993.
[128] K. Furukawa, D. G. Harrison, D. Saleh, H. Shennib, F. P. Chagnon, and A. Giaid, "Expression of nitric oxide synthase in the human nasal mucosa," *Am. J. Respir. Crit. Care Med.* vol. 153, n° 2, pp. 847-850, Feb. 1996, doi: 10.1164/ajrccm.153.2.8564142.
[129] J. M. Bernstein, "The molecular biology of nasal polyposis," *Curr. Allergy Asthma Rep.* vol. 1, n° 3, pp. 262-267, May 2001.
[130] F. Hiraide and H. Kakoi, "Histochemical study on innervation of glands and blood vessels in nasal polyps," *Acta Oto-Laryngol. Suppl.* vol. 430, p. 5-11, 1986.
[131] R. Jankowski, C. Rumeau, P. Gallet, and D. T. Nguyen, "Nasal polyposis (or chronic olfactory rhinitis)," *Ann. Fr. Oto-Rhino-Laryngol. Pathol. Cervico-Faciale*, vol. 135, n° 3, pp. 190-196, June 2018, doi: 10.1016/j.aforl.2017.09.014.
[132] Lundberg J, Lundberg J, Settergreen G, et al, "Nitric oxide, produced in theupper airways, may act in an "aerocrine" fashion to enhance pulmonary oxygenuptake in humans", *Acta Physiol Scand*, n° 155, pp. 467-8, 1995.
[133] R. Elsaesser and J. Paysan, "The sense of smell, its signalling pathways, and the dichotomy of cilia and microvilli in olfactory sensory cells", *BMC Neurosci.* vol. 8, n° 3, p. S1, Sept. 2007, doi: 10.1186/1471-2202-8-S3-S1.
[134] Hirschberg SR, "mitteilung über einen fall von nebenwirkung des aspirins", *Dtsch Med Wochenschr*, n° 28, p. 416, 1902.
[135] R. G. Slavin, "Relationship of nasal disease and sinusitis to bronchial asthma," *Ann. Allergy*, vol. 49, n° 2, pp. 76-79, August 1982.
[136] A. Szczeklik, "Clinical patterns of hypersensitivity to nonsteroidal anti-inflammatory drugs and their pathogenesis", *J ALLERGY CLIN IMMUNOL*, vol. 60, n° 5, p. 9, 1977.
[137] D. A. Moneret-Vautrin, M. Wayoff, and C. Bonne, "[Mechanisms of aspirin intolerance]," *Ann. Oto-Laryngol. Chir. Cervico Faciale Bull. Soc. Oto-Laryngol. Hopitaux Paris*, vol. 102, n° 5, p. 357-363, 1985.
[138] A. Szczeklik, R. J. Gryglewski, and G. Czerniawska-Mysik, "Relationship of inhibition of prostaglandin biosynthesis by analgesics to asthma attacks in aspirin-sensitive patients," *Br. Med. J.*, vol. 1, n° 5949, p. 67-69, Jan. 1975.

[139] A. Szczeklik, E. Niżankowska, M. Duplaga, and on behalf of the Aiane Investigators, "Natural history of aspirin-induced asthma," *Eur. Respir. J.*, vol. 16, n° 3, p. 432, Sept. 2000, doi: 10.1034/j.1399-3003.2000.016003432.x.
[140] P. Dessi and F. Facon, "Nasosinus polyposis in adults", *Encycl Méd Chir Oto-rhino-laryngologie*, p. 16, 2003.
[141] G. Brescia, C. Zanotti, D. Parrino, U. Barion, and G. Marioni, "Nasal polyposis pathophysiology: Endotype and phenotype open issues," *Am. J. Otolaryngol.* vol. 39, n° 4, pp. 441-444, August 2018, doi: 10.1016/j.amjoto.2018.03.020.
[142] K. E. Hulse, W. W. Stevens, B. K. Tan, and R. P. Schleimer, "Pathogenesis of nasal polyposis," *Clin. Exp. Allergy*, vol. 45, n° 2, pp. 328-346, Feb. 2015, doi: 10.1111/cea.12472.
[143] P. Borgeat and P. Sirois, "Leukotrienes: a major step in the understanding of immediate hypersensitivity reactions", *J. Med. Chem.* vol. 24, n° 2, pp. 121-126, Feb. 1981.
[144] M. C. Holroyde, R. E. Altounyan, M. Cole, M. Dixon, and E. V. Elliott, "Bronchoconstriction produced in man by leukotrienes C and D", *Lancet Lond. Engl.* vol. 2, n° 8236, pp. 17-18, July 1981.
[145] Safirstein BH, "Allergic bronchopulmonary aspergillosis with obstruction of the upper respiratory tract", *Chest*, n° 70, pp. 788-790, 1976.
[146] Katzenstein AL, Sale SR, Greenberger PA, "Allergic Aspergillus sinusitis: a newly recognized form of sinusitis", *J Allergy Clin Immunol*, n° 72, pp. 89-93, 1983.
[147] A. L. Katzenstein, S. R. Sale, and P. A. Greenberger, "Pathologic findings in allergic aspergillus sinusitis. A newly recognized form of sinusitis," *Am. J. Surg. Pathol.* vol. 7, n° 5, pp. 439-443, July 1983.
[148] Lamb D, Millar J, Johnston A., "Allergic aspergillus of the paranasal sinuses", *J Pathol*, n° 137, p. 56, 1982.
[149] Manning SC, Vuitch F, Weinberg AG, Brown OE, "Allergic aspergillosis: a newly recognized form of sinusitis in the pediatric population", *Laryngoscope*, vol. (7 Pt 1), n° 99, pp. 681-685, 1989.
[150] " Allergic Fungal Rhinosinusitis: Current Theories and Management Strategies - Marple - 2001 - The Laryngoscope - Wiley Online Library. " https://onlinelibrary.wiley.com/doi/abs/10.1097/00005537-200106000-00015 (accessed June 05, 2019).

Chapitre 7 : Pathological anatomy of polyps

The histopathology of nasosinusal polypoid tissue is varied, ranging from polypoid inflammatory conditions, to benign and malignant epithelial, mesenchymal tumors, and hemato-lymphoid neoplasms. In the context of chronic rhinosinusitis (CRS), polyp refers to benign, non-granulomatous inflammatory tissue projecting with epithelial duplication into the nasosinus cavity. There are several histopathological features that differentiate CRS nasal polyps from other types of polypoid lesions occurring in the nasosinus cavities. In addition, nasal polyps may have certain features of their own that distinguish them from the surrounding non-polypoid CRS mucosa.

7.1 Histopathology of polyps in CRS with polyps :

Approximately 20% of CRS patients have nasal polyps [151]. Histologically, polyps have been classified into several groups, according to the proposed etiology, the predominance of inflammatory cellular infiltration and the appearance of the stroma. This classification is purely descriptive and not specific to any associated disorder or underlying pathology.

7.1.1 Macroscopic appearance:

Macroscopically, most polyps are edematous, smooth and shiny with a soft consistency compared to the surrounding non-polypoid mucosa.

The cut surface is usually pale, edematous and translucent in appearance. Old, aged polyps may be white, firm and solid, suggesting extensive fibrosis. Polyps are usually mobile and often attached to the underlying mucosa by a sessile implantation base. The surrounding mucosa and middle turbinates are usually more erythematous and firm to palpation. During CRS, the mucosa may also appear polypoid, depending on the degree of edema, but without a sessile implant base. (**Figure 26**)

Polyps commonly arise from the middle meatus and sphenoethmoidal recess, and are often bilateral. However, unilateral polyps are not uncommon. Polyps vary in size, and in the most severe cases can completely fill the nasal cavity, even extending beyond the nostrils and choanae.

In long-standing polyps, the nasal bones may remodel, causing enlargement of the nasal pyramid. The mucosa of the middle turbinate, inferior turbinate, unciform process and nasal septum may also undergo polypoid degeneration.

Unlike the middle and upper turbinates, the anterior portion of the lower turbinate is rarely polypoid, and this may be due to the presence of squamous epithelium and aerodynamics in the region.

Generally, nasal polyps associated with CRS do not have a macroscopically ulcerated surface, and the presence of such a lesion may point to other pathologies. A lobulated or grape-like appearance may signify other pathologies such as nasosinusal inverted papilloma. However, based on appearance alone, the underlying pathology is not always possible to determine. Therefore, all polyps, especially unilateral ones, require histopathological examination.

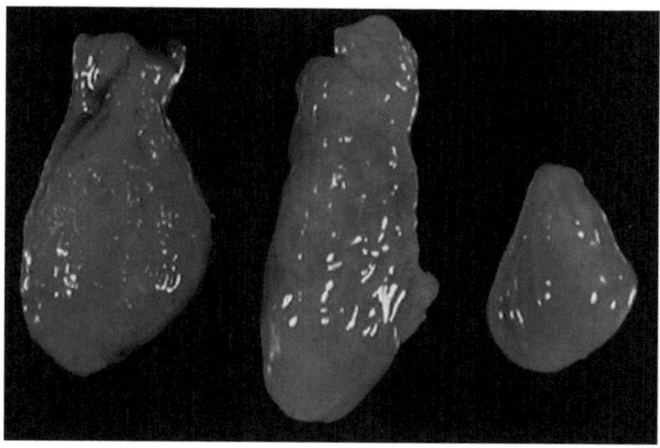

Figure 26*Macroscopic appearance of a series of edematous polyps. [10]*

7.1.2 Microscopic appearance:

The morphological appearance of polyps is non-specific, characterized by a varied inflammatory cellular infiltrate, rich or poor in eosinophils, connective tissue edema, thickening of the basement membrane and focal changes in the epithelium.

Secretory hyperplasia, with a preponderance of caliciform cells compared to ciliated cells, is most frequently observed.

In addition, alteration of the hair cells with abrasion of the basement membrane can be observed. These morphological changes in the polyp epithelium suggest changes in epithelial cell proliferation and differentiation related to polyp growth, local inflammation or in response to mechanical or other trauma. 9,62][

The main histological features of nasal polyps and mucosa in CRS compared to normal mucosa are the presence of structural changes involving the epithelium, submucosa and sometimes underlying bone, and the nature and degree of inflammatory cell infiltration.

Nasal polyps are usually lined with respiratory epithelium and have a basement membrane of variable thickness and an underlying stroma with a range of structural changes and inflammatory cells. Polyps have historically been classified according to their histological structural appearance and the nature of the predominant inflammatory cell population into: edematous polyps, eosinophilic or allergic polyps, chronic inflammatory polyps and seromucosal glandular polyps. The description eosinophilic and non-eosinophilic polyps is often used in the literature, but this classification is not specific to any associated or underlying pathology.

Edematous (**Figure 27**) and eosinophilic polyps are the most common type, and are also known as allergic nasal polyps. However, only a small proportion of CRS with polyps are associated with allergy.

In these, the polyps are lined with respiratory epithelium, with a range of mucosal alterations including ulceration, granulation tissue, epithelial and caliciform cellular hyperplasia and squamous metaplasia. The basement membrane is often thickened, with abundant submucosal edema.

Mucous retention cysts are common and vary in the amount of inflammatory cell infiltrate, which mainly contains scattered eosinophils, plasma cells and lymphocytes. Mucous glands are often present in the edematous polyp.

Edematous and eosinophilic polyps are found in all associated diseases, such as: eosinophilic mycotic CRS (EMCRS) , allergic fungal sinusitis, Fernand Widal triad, cystic fibrosis and Churg-Strauss syndrome.

Classically, nasal polyps associated with cystic fibrosis have a thin rather than thick basement membrane and less stromal eosinophilia, with more neutrophils, hence the name neutrophilic polyps, in addition to thick, eosinophil-rich mucus secretions.

The chronic inflammatory polyp (**Figure 28**), also known as the fibro-inflammatory polyp, is less common, forming less than 10% of inflammatory nasal polyps. It may present as an edematous polyp, or occasionally, when traumatized, the stroma may undergo secondary inflammatory remodeling resulting from myofibroblastic proliferation that may mimic a soft-tissue tumor. The main histological features are submucosal fibrosis and often a significant mixed inflammatory infiltrate, with lymphoid tissue predominating at the germinal centers. Like other nasal polyps, seromucosal glands are always present in the polyp, unlike true mesenchymal lesions, which tend to displace seromucosal glands. The surface epithelium is likely to show squamous metaplasia as a marker of chronicity.

Polyps with seromucosal gland hyperplasia are less common. Lesions in this category are relatively new and somewhat controversial as to their relationship to true epithelial tumors, including adenomatoid hamartoma of the respiratory epithelium and seromucosal hamartoma. 10,152-154][

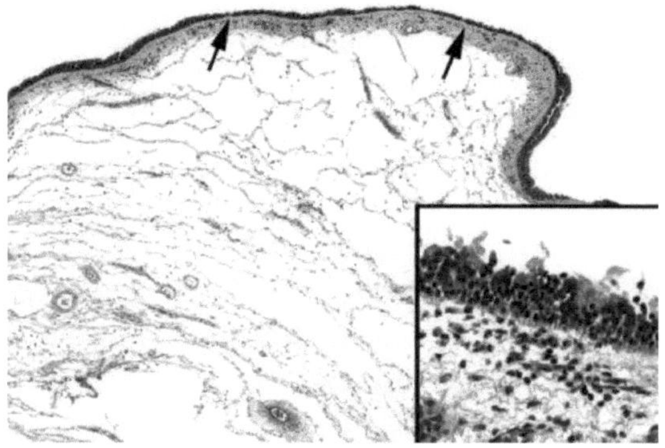

Figure 27*Edematous polyp.* [10]

(20 ×). This polyp shows a thickened basement membrane (arrows) and (400 ×). Marked submucosal edema.

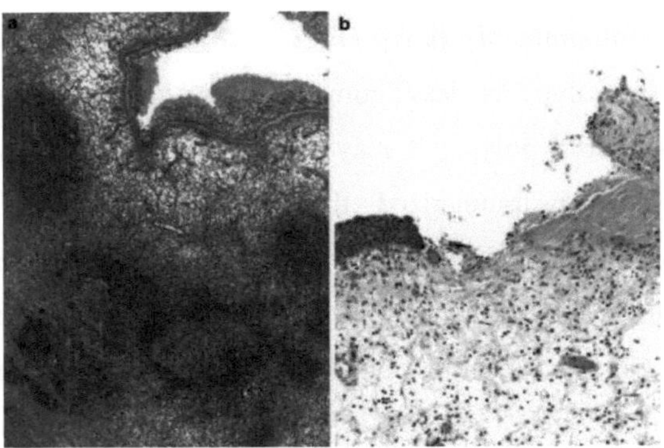

Figure 28*Chronic inflammatory polyps.* [10]

(a) (20 ×). This polyp shows exuberant lymphoid hyperplasia with germinal center reaction. (b) (100 ×). This polyp shows mucosal ulceration (right) and squamous metaplasia (left).

7.2 Histopathology of mucus:

A proportion of CRS with polyps also present a characteristically thick, dark and tenacious mucus, known as eosinophilic mucus (**Figure 29**). This mucus is usually found in allergic fungal sinusitis, but also in patients with severe and recalcitrant polypoid CRS, including cystic fibrosis, Fernand Widal disease and in the lungs of patients with allergic bronchopulmonary aspergillosis. [10]

Secretions associated with CRS with or without polyps have a range of consistencies and contain numerous inflammatory cells reflecting the infiltrate found in the mucosa and polyps. CRS secretions with polyps generally contain more eosinophils than those without, regardless of mucus consistency.

In the eosinophilic mycotic CRS group (EMCRS), secretions are typically thick and almost solid. This mucus typically shows clusters of eosinophils, eosinophil degradation products (Charcot Leyden crystals) and other inflammatory and epithelial cells. Fungal elements can be detected in 100% of these samples as silvery stains. This mucus, known as eosinophilic mucus, is the diagnostic criterion for EMCRS and allergic fungal sinusitis. [10]

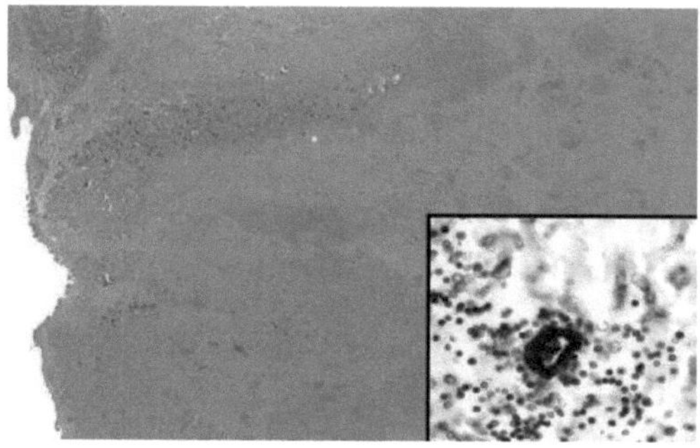

Figure 29*Allergic or "eosinophilic" mucus*. [10]

(40 ×). Intensely eosinophilic, bright pink granular appearance (Grocott's spot, 600 ×).

References :

[9] Peynegre, Freche, Fontanel, *la polypose naso sinusienne*. Société Française d'Oto-rhino-laryngologie et de Chirurgie de la Face et du Cou, 2000.

[10] T. M. Önerci and B. J. Ferguson, eds, *Nasal Polyposis: Pathogenesis, Medical and Surgical Treatment*. Berlin Heidelberg: Springer-Verlag, 2010. [62] G. A. Settipane, "Epidemiology of nasal polyps", *Allergy Asthma Proc.* vol. 17, n° 5, pp. 231-236, Oct. 1996.

[151] N. Bhattacharyya, "Clinical and symptom criteria for the accurate diagnosis of chronic rhinosinusitis", *The Laryngoscope*, vol. 116, n° 7 Pt 2 Suppl 110, p. 1-22, July 2006, doi: 10.1097/01.mlg.0000224508.59725.19.

[152] R. L. Werner and J. T. Castle, "Inflammatory Myofibroblastic Tumor of the Nasal Cavity," *Head Neck Pathol.* vol. 10, n° 3, pp. 336-339, Oct. 2015, doi: 10.1007/s12105-015-0662-9.

[153] B. M. Wenig and D. K. Heffner, "Respiratory epithelial adenomatoid hamartomas of the sinonasal tract and nasopharynx: a clinicopathologic study of 31 cases," *Ann. Otol. Rhinol. Laryngol.* vol. 104, n° 8, p. 639-645, August 1995, doi: 10.1177/000348949510400809.

[154] Y. F. Yilmaz, A. Titiz, M. Ozcan, M. S. Tezer, S. Ozlugedik, and A. Unal, "Bilateral antrochoanal polyps in an adult: a case report", *B-ENT*, vol. 3, n° 2, pp. 97-99, 2007.

Chapitre 8 : Clinical aspect [9,11,15,29,131,140]

8.1 Interrogation:

This is the key to diagnosis, and can be considered in several stages:

-Exposure: Exposure to occupational toxins, air conditioning and tobacco are systematically investigated, as they can influence the evolution of polyp disease.

-History: The patient's personal and family history of asthma, allergy and SNP is detailed.

-Disease history: This defines the onset of symptoms, their chronology and previous medical and surgical treatments.

- Age and gender: In the majority of cases, this pathology begins at the age of 40, most often in males, and is rare in children.

-Functional symptomatology: the reason for consultation is most often a lingering cold, with increasingly infrequent lulls, and the patient describes himself as a chronic cold sufferer. This is summed up in the acronym ADORE: A for anosmia, D for pain, O for obstruction, R for rhinorrhea and E for sneezing.

Anosmia - A: Olfactory disorders, which may be absent at first, range from simple hyposmia to anosmia. They are the main complaint of patients.

Facial pain - D: This is exceptional, except in the case of acute sinusitis or surgical complications (stenosis of the nasofrontal canal, mucocele).

They are of nasal or sinus projection and are most often just of the gravity type.

Their preferred location is the maxilla or midface.

Nasal obstruction - O: This may be absent at the start of the disease, but becomes increasingly pronounced as the disease progresses. It is then typically bilateral, permanent and increased in the supine position.

Rhinorrhea - R: Rhinorrhea is a symptom that varies in intensity, but is most often present on questioning. Apart from episodic superinfections, it is clear, bilateral and frequently posterior.

Sneezing - E: This indicates hyperreactivity of the nasal mucosa, and is manifested by bursts of sneezing.

8.2 Physical examination :

8.2.1 Inspection:

Examination should always begin with a thorough inspection of the nasal pyramid and sinus areas, looking for deformities suggestive of Woakes' polyposis deformans, polyps protruding through the nostril orifices, or surgical scars that could impose a differential diagnosis.

8.2.2 Palpation:

Involving the nasal pyramid and sinus areas, it can trigger pain, usually indicating an infectious complication.

8.2.3 Anterior rhinoscopy :

This is a speculum examination of the anterior part of the nasal cavity. It reveals the presence of polyps in both nasal cavities, which are usually bilateral, but may predominate on one side.

Polyps typically appear as translucent, pinkish-yellow grapes, sometimes with fine vascularization on their surface. Mucus appears stringy and thick, having lost its rheological characteristics.

8.2.4 Posterior rhinoscopy:

This is the laryngeal mirror examination of the cavum and choanae. It is increasingly being abandoned in favor of examination with flexible or rigid optics.

8.2.5 Endoscopic examination :

Nasal endoscopy is performed using a flexible fiberscope or, better still, a rigid 0° or 30° endoscope, depending on the practitioner's preference. This allows better image quality, and frees up one hand for palpation or sampling.

Examination must be meticulous, without preparation or after retraction of the nasal mucosa.

It is essential to gather information that includes evaluation of all the anatomical structures and regions of each nasal cavity, in search of constitutional abnormalities or those acquired through previous procedures; confirmation of the bilateral nature of the polyposis, since unilateral polyposis requires biopsies to rule out any tumoral development; and assessment of its extension, which is made easier by the use of different classifications based on the position of the polyps in relation to the structures of the middle meatus.

- **Three-dimensional classification**: [155]

It provides information on the location of polyps in all three planes of space.

- Horizontally, polyps are classified as follows:

H0: no polyp.
H1: polyp limited to the middle meatus.
H2: polyp extending beyond the middle meatus without reaching the nasal septum.

HT: polyp extending beyond the middle meatus and reaching the nasal septum.

-The polyps are classified vertically:

V0: no polyp.
V1: polyp in the middle meatus only.
VI: polyp extending down the middle meatus beyond the upper edge of the inferior turbinate.
VS: polyp extending above the middle meatus, between the septum and middle turbinate.
VT: polyp occupying the entire vertical plane of the nasal cavity.

-The polyps are classified anteroposteriorly:

P0: no polyp.
P1: polyps in the middle meatus only.
PA: polyps extending anterior to the middle meatus, touching the head of the inferior turbinate.
PP: polyps extending behind the middle meatus, touching the tail of the inferior turbinate.
PT: polyps occupying the entire anteroposterior plane of the nasal cavity.

- **Rouvier's classification**: [156]

- stage 0: normal mucosa.
- stage 1: edema or tiny polyp.
- stage 2: polyposis not extending beyond the lower edge of the middle turbinate.
- stage 3: polyposis affecting the back of the lower cornet.
- stage 4: obstructive or almost obstructive polyposis.

- **The French ENT Society classification**: [140]

This is the most common and easiest to use in practice, and we use this classification with all our patients.

- stage 1: polyps located in the middle meatus.
- stage 2: polyps developed in the nasal cavity but not extending beyond the upper limit of the inferior turbinate.
- stage 3: polyps reaching the floor of the nasal cavity.

Other classifications based on polyp schematization have been proposed, as reported by Johansson, who evaluated five methods of polyp staging, and demonstrated that evaluation by lateral imaging, nasal cavity patency and Lildholdt's method gave almost identical results by several examiners, and nasal obstruction was not a good indicator of polyp size. He also found in another work that diagrammatic reproduction of polyps is the method that allows detection of changes in polyp size after use of topical corticoids. [157]

8.2.6 The rest of the ENT and general examination:

The aim is to evaluate the impact of this polyposis pathology, and to look for other associated diseases that may aggravate the evolution of polyposis or limit its medical or surgical management.

8.2.7 Quality of life tests :

Using quality of life questionnaires, we can assess the degree of discomfort as experienced by the patient, giving a precise idea of the quality of life associated with their SNP, even before considering any medical or surgical treatment.

8.3 Additional tests :

8.3.1 Pneumo-allergological workup : [9,11,158-160]

A pneumo-allergological inventory is essential at this stage, to assess the presence of overt asthma, detect latent bronchial hyperreactivity and look for atopic conditions.

Phadiatop, skin tests for type I hypersensitivity and a EFR with a metacholine test are performed according to specialist opinion.

Any history of intolerance to aspirin, NSAIDs, preservatives or food colorings leads us to suspect that the patient is intolerant.

-Skin tests: Skin reactivity to allergens in the atopic patient is an excellent reflection of nasal reactivity. Although a positive response to skin tests does not necessarily imply the existence of an allergy, these tests are highly accurate and reliable if carried out in a standardized way.

-Eosinophil count: very high counts above 1500/dl point to a particular etiology, sometimes allergic, but also non-allergic, as in the case of parasitosis.

-Total IgE assay: Although total IgE levels are usually high, normal or even low levels do not rule out atopy. Total IgE levels are no longer of great value in the diagnosis of allergy.

Multi-allergen screening tests: These are serum tests, such as Phadiatop, which detect specific IgE antibodies in the patient's serum, directed against the most common pneumallergens. These tests are qualitative, not quantitative, with a positive or negative response, but their specificity and sensitivity are in excess of 80-90%.

Specific serum IgE assays: These are a valuable adjunct to skin testing, but should not be used as a first-line or routine measure. They are useful when there is a discrepancy between clinical data on the suspected allergen and the results of skin tests, or when the latter cannot be performed. These tests have the advantage of being risk-free for the patient, with no false positives, and are not influenced by medication intake, but they are expensive and take some time to obtain results.

-Aspirin oral provocation test: In practice, any history of intolerance to aspirin, NSAIDs or food preservatives or colorings leads us to suspect and consider the patient as intolerant, and makes it dangerous to perform these tests.

-Nasal provocation tests: These are not commonly used, and are reserved for very specific situations.

Other biological tests: such as analysis of basophil activation markers (CD63) or eosinophils, which are currently being validated, or analysis of nasal secretions or sputum showing hyper-eosinophilia, which is not specific to allergic pathology.

If a surgical procedure is planned, a preoperative work-up may be requested, including a blood count, a renal work-up and a characterization of the patient's blood type.

-Respiratory function tests (RFTs): These show reversible bronchial obstruction under beta-2 mimetics, characteristic of asthma. Its purpose is to detect obstructive syndrome or bronchial hyperreactivity in the context of SFN.

8.3.2 Radiological and imaging work-up : [9,10,15,140,158]

8.3.2.1 Standard sinus radiographs:

Classically, three incidences are performed: a high-face incidence (forehead-nose-plate), a Blondeau incidence (nose-chin-plate) and a Hirtz incidence (patient supine, vertex against the table, Virchow plane parallel to the table). In fact, they are of limited interest, as they do not study the ethmoid, sphenoid and ostiomental region well enough to highlight complications, and do not provide the surgeon with complete anatomical precision.

CT scans should be avoided because of their low diagnostic efficacy, high radiation exposure and high cost.

8.3.2.2 Computed tomography (CT) : [161-165]

Morphological assessment is dominated by computed tomography (CT), today's gold standard for exploring the nasosinus cavities, performed in high-resolution mode with spiral acquisitions and contrast-free axial, coronal and sagittal reconstructions in bone windows.

Considered the indication of choice for SNPs for the following reasons:

- It determines the extent of polyposis and the response to medical treatment;

- it explores cases of atypical polyposis, enabling a differential diagnosis to be made;

- it highlights the existence of nasosinus anatomical anomalies;

- it looks for pre- or post-operative complications;

- it guides the surgical procedure to be performed;

- it assesses postoperative recurrence;

- it is considered to have medicolegal value [166].

Numerous classifications exist in the Anglo-Saxon literature, including those of **Lund and** Mackay [167] is internationally recognized, and enables a CT score to be assigned to the patient, thus facilitating follow-up and assessment of recurrences:

- Sine analysis :

- Score 0: healthy sinus.
- Score 1: partial opacity.
- Score 2: total opacity.

- Analysis of the middle meatus:

- Score 0: ostio-meatal complex permeable.
- Score 2: dyspermeable ostio-meatal complex.

Each sinus is scored on the right and left: maxillary, anterior ethmoidal, posterior ethmoidal, frontal, sphenoidal; and the ostio-meatal complex on the right and left. The sum of all ratings is 0 to 24. [167[167-170]

It must be stressed that a sinus opacity is not synonymous with a polyp, but may indicate simple retention.

Anatomical variations can be encountered, we mainly mention :

- Spontaneous dehiscence of the papyraceous lamina: always unilateral, these dehiscences are characterized by a veritable herniation of the orbital contents into the ethmoidal cavity. They are generally confined to the anterior ethmoid, and occur in less than 1% of cases. Such abnormalities may be confused with the diagnosis of ethmoidal sinusitis, and are all the more difficult to recognize when associated with chronic sinus pathology. [171]

- Differences in height between the two roofs of the lateral masses of the ethmoid: Such variations occur in 10% of cases. The right ethmoid roof is eight times out of ten lower than the left, with a difference of up to 7 mm. It is interesting to compare these findings with the fact that the surgical complications described by several authors appear with a significant difference more frequently on the right side than on the left. Although these authors have incriminated the discomfort felt by a right-handed surgeon operating on a right side, the difference in height of the ethmoidal roofs, with the right roof lower than the left, making it vulnerable during the surgical act remains an attractive hypothesis. [172]

A classification system has been developed to help predict the surgical risks associated with this difference in height. In 1962, Keros defined three categories in his classification (**Figure 30**) [173,174] :

-type **I (**1-3 mm, 26.3% of the population),
-type **II** (4-7mm 73.3% of the population),
-type **III** (8-16mm 0.5% of the population).

- **Intrasphenoidal procidences of the internal carotid artery:** Their incidence varies between 12% and 25% of sphenoidal sinuses examined. In 10% of cases, the internal carotid artery protrudes over more than half its circumference. This makes it particularly vulnerable to surgical injury. A thin protective lamina of bone more than 1 mm thick surrounding the internal carotid artery has been demonstrated, making its injury in gentle hands rare. [175[175-177]

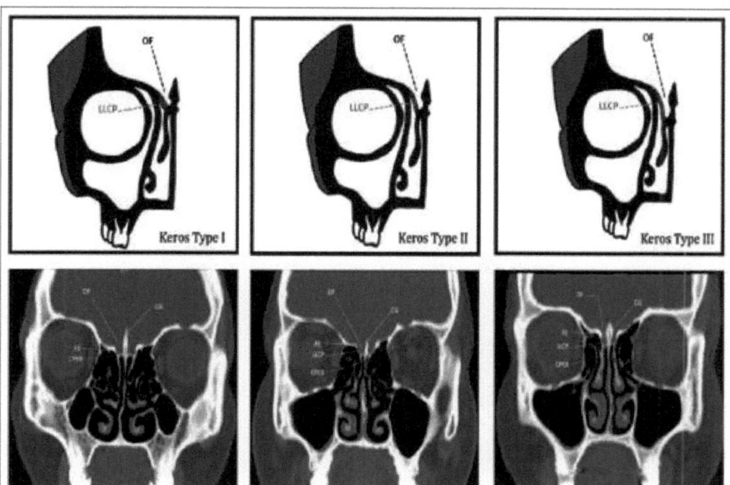

Figure 30*Schematic representation and coronal CT sections showing the three types of the Keros classification.* [178]

(CG: Crista galli, OF: Fossette Olfactive, FE: Fovea ethmoidalis, LLCP: Lame Latérale du toit de l'éthmoïde, CPEB: La lame Criblée de l'éthmoïde).

- Optic nerve protrusion into the sphenoid sinus: In 8% of cases, the optic nerve protrudes into the sphenoid cavity over an area of at least half its circumference. Usually unilateral, but sometimes this procidence may be bilateral and then associated with dehiscence of both internal carotids. [178]

8.3.2.3 Magnetic resonance imaging (MRI) : [166,179]

It has no diagnostic value, other than as a differential diagnosis in the case of atypical presentation or suspicion, and is also useful for assessing complications.

References :

[9] Peynegre, Freche, Fontanel, *la polypose naso sinusienne*. Société Française d'Oto-rhino-laryngologie et de Chirurgie de la Face et du Cou, 2000.

[10] T. M. Önerci and B. J. Ferguson, eds, *Nasal Polyposis: Pathogenesis, Medical and Surgical Treatment*. Berlin Heidelberg: Springer-Verlag, 2010.

[11] Mahassine EL HARRAS, "la polypose nasosinusienne: place de la chirurgie endonasale", Université CADI AYYAD, Marrakech, 2011.

[15] SOULTANA RABIE, "nasosinusal polyposis: experience of the ENT department at Moulay Ismail Hospital in Meknes (à propos de 60 cas)", Université Sidi Mohammed ben Abdellah, FES, 2015.

[29] R. Jankowski, *Du dysfonctionnement naso-sinusien chronique au dysfonctionnement ostio-meatal*. Paris: Société Française d'Oto-rhino-laryngologie et de Chrurgie de la Face et du Cou, 2006.

[131] R. Jankowski, C. Rumeau, P. Gallet, and D. T. Nguyen, "Nasal polyposis (or chronic olfactory rhinitis)," *Ann. Fr. Oto-Rhino-Laryngol. Pathol. Cervico-Faciale*, vol. 135, n° 3, pp. 190-196, June 2018, doi: 10.1016/j.aforl.2017.09.014.

[140] P. Dessi and F. Facon, "Nasosinus polyposis in adults", *Encycl Méd Chir Oto-rhino-laryngologie*, p. 16, 2003.

[155] M. C. A. de Sousa, H. M. G. Becker, C. G. Becker, M. Moreira de Castro, N. J. Alves de Sousa, and R. E. dos S. Guimarães, "Reproducibility of the three-dimensional endoscopic staging system for nasal polyposis," *Braz. J. Otorhinolaryngol*, vol. 75, n° 6, pp. 814-820, Nov. 2009, doi: 10.1016/S1808-8694(15)30542-5.

[156] Rouvier P, Vandeventer G, El hkoury J, De Lanversion H., "Les résultats à long terme (sur 5 ans) de l'éthmoïdectomie dans la polypose invalidante", *J Fr ORL*, vol. 2, n° 40, p. 102-105, 1991.

[157] L. Johansson, K. Holmberg, I. Melén, P. Stierna, and M. Bende, "Sensitivity of a new grading system for studying nasal polyps with the potential to detect early changes in polyp size after treatment with a topical corticosteroid (budesonide)," *Acta Otolaryngol. (Stockh.)*, vol. 122, n° 1, pp. 49-53, Jan. 2002.

[158] Freche Ch, Fantanel JP, *L'obstruction nasale*, Arnette Blackwell. Paris: Société Française d'Oto-rhino-laryngologie et de Chirurgie de la Face et du Cou, 1996.

[159] A. Didier, J. Percodani, Doussau S., and E. Serrano, "Rhinite allergique : démarche diagnostique", *Rev fr Allergol*, n° 7, p. 602-609, 1998.

[160] M. Raffard and H. Partouche, "Allergologie en pratique", *EMC - Traité Médecine AKOS*, vol. 3, n° 1, p. 1-9, Jan. 2008, doi: 10.1016/S1634-6939(07)32304-1.
[161] S. Chaouir, A. Hanine, T. Amic, A. Abrouq, and M. B. Ameur, "Les polyposes naso-sinusiennes. Apport de la tomodensitométrie. A propos de 41 cas ", p. 5, 2001.
[162] D. F. Jiannetto and M. F. Pratt, "Correlation between preoperative computed tomography and operative findings in functional endoscopic sinus surgery", *The Laryngoscope*, vol. 105, n° 9 Pt 1, pp. 924-927, Sept. 1995, doi: 10.1288/00005537-199509000-00010.
[163] G. A. Lloyd, V. J. Lund, and G. K. Scadding, "CT of the paranasal sinuses and functional endoscopic surgery: a critical analysis of 100 symptomatic patients," *J. Laryngol. Otol.* vol. 105, n° 3, pp. 181-185, March 1991.
[164] F. Meloni, F. Stomeo, and C. Bozzo, "[Coronal CT in the indication of the endoscopic surgery of the sinus]", *Acta Otorhinolaryngol. Ital. Organo Uff. Della Soc. Ital. Otorinolaringol. E Chir. Cerv.-facc.*, vol. 15, n° 3, pp. 214-218, June 1995.
[165] R. J. Witte, J. V. Heurter, D. F. Orton, and F. J. Hahn, "Limited axial CT of the paranasal sinuses in screening for sinusitis," *AJR Am. J. Roentgenol*, vol. 167, n° 5, pp. 1313-1315, Nov. 1996, doi: 10.2214/ajr.167.5.8911203.
[166] M. Re, G. Magliulo, R. Romeo, F. M. Gioacchini, and E. Pasquini, "Risks and medico-legal aspects of endoscopic sinus surgery: a review," *Eur. Arch. Oto-Rhino-Laryngol. Off. J. Eur. Fed. Oto-Rhino-Laryngol. Soc. EUFOS Affil. Ger. Soc. Oto-Rhino-Laryngol. - Head Neck Surg.* vol. 271, n° 8, pp. 2103-2117, August 2014, doi: 10.1007/s00405-013-2652-4.
[167] V. J. Lund and I. S. Mackay, "Staging in rhinosinusitus", *Rhinology*, vol. 31, n° 4, pp. 183-184, Dec. 1993.
[168] L. Boari and N. P. de Castro Júnior, "Diagnosis of chronic rhinosinusitis in patients with cystic fibrosis: correlation between anamnesis, nasal endoscopy and computed tomography", *Rev. Bras. Otorrinolaringol.* vol. 71, n° 6, pp. 705-710, Dec. 2005, doi: 10.1590/S0034-72992005000600003.
[169] C. Hopkins, J. P. Browne, R. Slack, V. Lund, and P. Brown, "The Lund-Mackay staging system for chronic rhinosinusitis: how is it used and what does it predict?", *Otolaryngol.--Head Neck Surg. Off. J. Am. Acad. Otolaryngol.-Head Neck Surg.* vol. 137, n° 4, pp. 555-561, Oct. 2007, doi: 10.1016/j.otohns.2007.02.004.
[170] V. J. Lund and D. W. Kennedy, "Staging for rhinosinusitis," *Otolaryngol.--Head Neck Surg. Off. J. Am. Acad. Otolaryngol.-Head Neck Surg.* vol. 117, n° 3 Pt 2, p. S35-40, Sept. 1997, doi: 10.1016/S0194-59989770005-6.

[171] G. Moulin *et al*, "Dehiscence of the lamina papyracea of the ethmoid bone: CT findings," *Am. J. Neuroradiol.* vol. 15, n° 1, pp. 151-153, Jan. 1994.
[172] P. Dessi, G. Moulin, J. M. Triglia, M. Zanaret, and M. Cannoni, "Difference in the height of the right and left ethmoidal roofs: a possible risk factor for ethmoidal surgery. Prospective study of 150 CT scans", *J. Laryngol. Otol.* vol. 108, n° 3, pp. 261-262, March 1994.
[173] A. Skorek, D. Tretiakow, T. Szmuda, and T. Przewozny, "Is the Keros classification alone enough to identify patients with the "dangerous ethmoid"? An anatomical study", *Acta Otolaryngol (Stockh.)*, vol. 137, n° 2, pp. 196-201, Feb. 2017, doi: 10.1080/00016489.2016.1225316.
[174] P. Gupta and R. P, "RADIOLOGICAL OBSERVATION OF ETHMOID ROOF ON BASIS OF KEROS CLASSIFICATION AND ITS APPLICATION IN ENDONASAL SURGERY," *Int. J. Anat. Res.* vol. 5, n° 3.2, pp. 4204-4207, August 2017, doi: 10.16965/ijar.2017.284.
[175] P. Dessi, G. Moulin, J. M. Bartoli, and M. Cannoni, "[Intra-sphenoidal prolapse of the internal carotid artery. Computed tomography of 300 sinuses]", *Presse Medicale Paris Fr. 1983*, vol. 23, n° 13, pp. 616-617, Apr. 1994.
[176] P. A. Hudgins, "Complications of endoscopic sinus surgery. The role of the radiologist in prevention", *Radiol. Clin. North Am.* vol. 31, n° 1, pp. 21-32, Jan. 1993.
[177] J. Kainz and H. Stammberger, "Danger Areas of the Posterior Rhinobasis: An Endoscopic and Anatomical-surgical Study", *Acta Otolaryngol. (Stockh.)*, vol. 112, n° 5, pp. 852-861, Jan. 1992, doi: 10.3109/00016489209137484.
[178] P. Dessi, G. Moulin, F. Castro, C. Chagnaud, and M. Cannoni, "Protrusion of the optic nerve into the ethmoid and sphenoid sinus: prospective study of 150 CT studies," *Neuroradiology*, vol. 36, n° 7, pp. 515-516, Oct. 1994.
[179] C. Ide, J. P. Trigaux, and P. Eloy, "Chronic sinusitis: the role of imaging", *Acta Otorhinolaryngol. Belg.* vol. 51, n° 4, pp. 247-258, 1997.

Chapitre 9 : Clinical forms

Because of its associations and pathophysiological mechanisms, SNP is a pathology that can occur in isolation or in syndromes.

Various types of SNP have been described [140] :

- type I: isolated polyposis ;
- type II: polyposis associated with asthma ;
- type III or Widal triad: combining asthma and intolerance to aspirin;
- type IV or unclassifiable: Woakes syndrome, Young's syndrome, ciliary dyskinesia or cystic fibrosis.

9.1 Typical shape:

This is a previously described case of bilateral polyposis in young adults (see clinical aspect).

9.2 Associated nasal forms :

9.2.1 Nasal polyposis associated with sinus opacities:

Opacities of the maxillary, frontal or sphenoid sinuses are very common on nasal polyposis CT scans, and vary in presentation from one sinus to another and from one patient to another. They reflect an associated pathology of the paranasal sinuses [131] :

-An opacity suggestive of an ordinary sinus serous cyst may have no impact on the management of polyposis;

-An opacity suggestive of framed hypertrophy of the mucosa does not a priori interfere with NO production, but merits a limited procedure that preserves ostial function;

-An opacity suggestive of retained secretions may lead to aspiration through the natural ostium to determine the nature of the secretions:

seromucous, purulent, or sometimes with a firm, sticky consistency, requiring an endoscopic procedure for evacuation and washing;

-A complete opacity of the sinus does not allow us to prejudge its nature;

-an associated opacity suggestive of a sinus fungal bullet may lead to a surgical decision.

9.2.2 Nasal polyposis associated with olfactory cleft hamartoma:

Adenomatoid respiratory epithelial hamartomas (HERA) are rare, benign glandular proliferations of the nasal cavity and nasopharynx, first described as a specific clinico-pathological entity by Wenig and Heffner in 1995 [153]. In this original characterization, 70% of HERAs presented with isolated involvement of the nasal cavity, the posterior septum being the most frequent site of origin. In addition, imaging evidence of expansion into the olfactory cleft implicated it as a potential site of origin rather than the nasal septum.

Macroscopically, HERAs presented as edematous, pinkish-yellow masses with a shiny surface similar to that of inflammatory polyps but generally darker, with an indurated, rubbery consistency.

A hamartoma should be suspected if the olfactory cleft is opacified and enlarged on CT. Not all polyps developed in the olfactory cleft are hamartomas; only histology can confirm the diagnosis, provided that suspicious polyps are separated for anatomopathological analysis. [153,180-183]

9.2.3 Nasal polyposis with deviated septum:

Septal deviation can be a factor aggravating nasal obstruction or representing a relative obstacle to local therapeutics, and can impede endoscope access during nasal polyposis surgery.

9.2.4 Nasal polyposis associated with allergic rhinitis:

Only the clinical manifestations of seasonal allergic rhinitis, which very often began in adolescence even before the development of polyposis, and are added seasonally to the perennial symptoms of polyposis, can be easily diagnosed, by the aggravation of the usual clinical symptomatology. [67]

9.3 Associated respiratory and systemic forms:

9.3.1 Nasal polyposis and asthma:

The association of PNS with asthma is classic. It is exceptional in children, and the average age of diagnosis of polyposis in an asthmatic patient is around 30-50 years.

In around two-thirds of cases, polyposis is diagnosed after the onset of asthma, often late in the course of bronchial symptoms. This observation may be explained by the patient's neglect of nasal symptoms, which often begin insidiously.

Although polyposis is not included in international guidelines for the management of asthmatic disease, in daily practice it is often considered a destabilizing factor, and some authors point to the improvement in bronchial symptomatology and the reduction in exacerbation of attacks after management of SFN. [9,184,185]

9.3.2 Polyposis and intolerance to aspirin and NSAIDs:

Clinical manifestations are either cutaneous or respiratory in nature, typically occurring not immediately, but on average an hour and a half after ingestion.

Respiratory intolerance is expressed by symptoms such as nasal obstruction followed by rhinorrhea, conjunctival hyperhemia giving the appearance of Russian rabbit eyes, most often preceded by an expiratory cough or even an asthma attack, which can lead to a serious or even fatal acute attack.

Angioedema is the most common expression of the cutaneous form, unlike isolated acute urticaria, which is rare. [9,184]

9.3.3 Fernand Widal (or Samter) triad:

Combining nasosinusal polyposis, intrinsic asthma, and intolerance to aspirin and NSAIDs [78]. It occurs in both men and women, usually in their fifties, is rare in adolescence and exceptional in childhood.

SFN is characterized by the disability of nasal obstruction and anosmia, the relative importance of signs of associated nasal hyperreactivity, such as rhinorrhea and pituitary mucosal dysesthesias. [140]

Endoscopically and tomodensitometrically, there is no difference with other types of SNP. [9].

This asthma is characterized by its late onset and non-allergic character, and is severe or severe in around 70% of cases, compared with 30% of mild or intermittent cases. Bronchoalveolar lavage of the bronchial mucosa reveals frank eosinophilia. [9,186]

Recurrent ENT or bronchial respiratory infections are frequently found, sometimes preceding the onset of the triad. [187]

The diagnosis of Widal's disease is made on the basis of clinical symptoms and intolerance to aspirin and NSAIDs.

9.3.4 Tetrad:

This is the association between the triad described above and chronic seromucous otitis. The onset of seromucosal otitis probably results from the spread of inflammatory pathology to all the cavities formed by pneumatization and could be accompanied by a generalized alteration in NO production. [188[188-190]

9.4 Unilateral and asymmetrical nasal polyposis:

Unilateral nasal polyposis with healthy contralateral ethmoid on CT is suspected of being tumoral, masked by sentinel edematous polyps. On the other hand, unilateral nasal polyposis of any stage with pathological contralateral ethmoid on CT may be asymmetric polyposis.

Certain anatomical conditions predispose to this type of polyposis, such as septal deviations, hypertrophy of the inferior cornet, and concha bullosa. [9,131]

9.5 Polyposis and fungal sinusitis:

This syndrome is presented as a particular form of non-invasive, extra-mucosal fungal sinusitis in young immunocompetent subjects, regardless of sex. Asthma is present in 40-80% of cases, nasal polyposis resistant to several medical and surgical treatments in 90-100%, and atopy in 40-80%. [88,89,191,192]

Radiologically, CT scans most often show multisinus involvement, with the presence of heterogeneous opacities with areas of calcification and, in 20% of cases, erosions. [193,194]

On magnetic resonance imaging, it shows a central hyposignal in T1 and T2, which increases in the periphery. [195,196]

Direct mycological examination after staining with Gomori Grocott reveals mycelial filaments, and culture on Sabouraud media identifies the fungus involved, dominated by the Dematiae family. [197,198]

Intraoperative macroscopic appearance shows thick, viscous, greenish secretions with a "putty" appearance. [199]

Anatomopathological examination of this material confirms the diagnosis, demonstrating the classic appearance of allergic mucin consisting of altered polynuclear aggregates, Charcot-Leyden crystals and altered mycelial filaments. [89]

Diagnostic criteria have been proposed by Bent and Kuhn [86] :

- notion of type I hypersensitivity;
- nasosinus polyposis ;
- radiographic criteria ;
- mucus rich in eosinophils and fungal elements without tissue invasion.

9.6 Nasal polyposis in children and young adults:

Nasal polyposis is usually diagnosed in adulthood. If it occurs before the age of 18, cystic fibrosis, primary ciliary dyskinesia or immune deficiency should be investigated. These forms are the nasal expression of a mucus disease in the case of cystic fibrosis, or a cilia disease in the case of ciliary dyskinesia. Associated bronchopulmonary manifestations are of a chronic infectious nature.

9.6.1 PNS and cystic fibrosis:

Cystic fibrosis is an autosomal recessive inherited disorder of the exocrine glands, characterized by thick, viscous secretions in multiple body systems, including the sinuses, upper and lower respiratory tracts. Its incidence is high in the Caucasian population, affecting 1/ 2,500 live births in the USA. [200]

It is incriminated in the majority of polyposis cases in children. This association with polyposis was demonstrated by Bodian and then Lurie in 1957. [140]

The incidence of PNS in this condition varies from series to series. Triglia [201] reported a polyposis incidence of 54.8% in an evaluation of 135 patients with cystic fibrosis, representing 72% of all SNPs diagnosed in children. Peak incidence occurs between 4 and 12 years of age [202].

The association of polyposis and cystic fibrosis in its classic form with pulmonary involvement, pancreatic insufficiency and elevated sweat chloride is found in 6 to 50% of cases [201,203].

The etiopathogenesis of SFN in cystic fibrosis is still poorly understood, with genetics remaining a definite factor, and Pseudomonas colonization and allergy yet to be confirmed. [10]

Clinically, the functional manifestations of PNS are non-specific. They associate nasal obstruction, rhinorrhea, sneezing, anosmia and facial pain evolving in a chronic mode. [204]

On examination, the polyps have a classic appearance; it is the presence of greenish mucopurulent secretions due to pyocyanic superinfection that should raise suspicion of cystic fibrosis. [10]

The evolution of SNP is difficult to assess, and spontaneous regression is rare. Antibiotic therapy helps to control infectious outbreaks, and to cover the associated corticosteroid therapy. Surgical control is most often required, either through polypectomy or a more extensive procedure opening up all the sinuses.

9.6.2 PNS and primary ciliary dyskinesia syndrome:

Primitive ciliary dyskinesia is a pathology related to an abnormality in the constitution of the cilia (absence of dynein arms); it leads to a disorder in mucociliary purification. In 50% of cases, this is Kartagener's syndrome, which combines situs inversus, bronchiectasis and chronic rhinosinus pathology. Transmission is autosomal recessive. Diagnosis is made after study of the ciliary beat. [205]

The frequency of polyposis in ciliary pathology is poorly understood, estimated at between 0 and 25% and as high as 68%. [205[205-207]

Clinically, it presents as recurrent or chronic airway infections, starting in the first months of life and associating with infertility in adulthood. In some cases, a classic-appearing PNS may be associated. [140]

Phase-contrast light microscopy and electron microscopy of a sample of epithelial cells collected by brushing the nasal mucosa, provides a precise etiological diagnosis.

The therapeutic management of SNP in these patients follows the same rules as for primary polyposis.

9.6.3 Woakes disease:

Woakes syndrome was first described in 1885, by Dr. E. Woakes in connection with a case, as necrotizing ethmoiditis with nasal polyps and nasal enlargement [208].

In 1923, the Société Française de Laryngologie defined the syndrome with four characteristics [209] bilateral nasal polyps in the middle meatus, beginning in childhood, ethmoiditis, hypertrophic and deforming process of the nasal pyramid and therapeutic failure with constant and rapid recurrences.

The etiopathogenesis of this syndrome remains unknown. Various authors have discussed genetic factors, an infectious origin, mainly syphilitic, or even external noxious agents and allergies, accelerating polyp growth. 210,211][

However, in many cases, no agent or allergy could be found. This confirms that this syndrome is only a clinical entity. [212,213]

This is a PNS that is particularly resistant to medical or surgical treatment, with multiple recurrences. The deformity rarely requires rhinoplasty.

9.6.4 Idiopathic PNS in children:

In the event of a blank etiological workup, the diagnosis of idiopathic nasal polyposis in children can be accepted, and a management plan similar to that for adults can be proposed. [214[214-216]

9.7 PNS for older subjects:

It does not differ from the type of description in young people.

9.8 Non-allergic eosinophilic rhinitis (NARES):

NARES is characterized by a syndrome of nasal hyperreactivity, without association with any allergic factor, with constant eosinophilia of nasal secretions. [217] Clinical and scanographic symptoms, are those of typical polyposis, but without visualization of polyps in endoscopy. [218]

The diagnosis of NARES is made on the basis of an eosinophilia greater than 20% on cytology of nasal secretions. If eosinophilia is less than 20%, the presence of fluctuations or a reduced sense of smell raise suspicion of NARES. [219]

The seriousness of NARES lies in its potential to develop into nasal polyposis or Fernand Widal syndrome. [220]

In the light of evo-devo conceptions, the transformation of the term NARES into NAORES (Non-allergic olfactory rhinitis with eosinophilia syndrome) would be justified. [131]

References :

[9] Peynegre, Freche, Fontanel, *la polypose naso sinusienne*. Société Française d'Oto-rhino-laryngologie et de Chirurgie de la Face et du Cou, 2000.

[10] T. M. Önerci and B. J. Ferguson, eds, *Nasal Polyposis: Pathogenesis, Medical and Surgical Treatment*. Berlin Heidelberg: Springer-Verlag, 2010.

[67] P. K. Keith *et al*, "Nasal polyps: effects of seasonal allergen exposure", *J. Allergy Clin. Immunol*, vol. 93, n° 3, pp. 567-574, March 1994.

[86] J. P. Bent and F. A. Kuhn, "Diagnosis of allergic fungal sinusitis," *Otolaryngol.--Head Neck Surg. Off. J. Am. Acad. Otolaryngol.-Head Neck Surg*. vol. 111, n° 5, pp. 580-588, Nov. 1994, doi: 10.1177/019459989411100508.

[88] J. P. Corey, "Allergic fungal sinusitis," *Otolaryngol. Clin. North Am*. vol. 25, n° 1, pp. 225-230, Feb. 1992.

[89] S. C. Manning and M. Holman, "Further evidence for allergic pathophysiology in allergic fungal sinusitis", *The Laryngoscope*, vol. 108, n° 10, pp. 1485-1496, Oct. 1998.

[131] R. Jankowski, C. Rumeau, P. Gallet, and D. T. Nguyen, "Nasal polyposis (or chronic olfactory rhinitis)," *Ann. Fr. Oto-Rhino-Laryngol. Pathol. Cervico-Faciale*, vol. 135, n° 3, pp. 190-196, June 2018, doi: 10.1016/j.aforl.2017.09.014.

[140] P. Dessi and F. Facon, "Nasosinus polyposis in adults", *Encycl Méd Chir Oto-rhino-laryngologie*, p. 16, 2003.

[153] B. M. Wenig and D. K. Heffner, "Respiratory epithelial adenomatoid hamartomas of the sinonasal tract and nasopharynx: a clinicopathologic study of 31 cases," *Ann. Otol. Rhinol. Laryngol.* vol. 104, n° 8, p. 639-645, August 1995, doi: 10.1177/000348949510400809.

[180] L. N. al et, "Respiratory adenomatoid hamartoma must be suspected on CT-scan enlargement of the olfactory clefts. - PubMed - NCBI." https://www.ncbi.nlm.nih.gov/pubmed/17216743 (accessed June 17, 2019).

[181] D. T. Nguyen, G. Gauchotte, F. Arous, J.-M. Vignaud, and R. Jankowski, "Respiratory epithelial adenomatoid hamartoma of the nose: an updated review," *Am. J. Rhinol. Allergy*, vol. 28, n° 5, pp. 187-192, Oct. 2014, doi: 10.2500/ajra.2014.28.4085.

[182] C. Delbrouck, S. Fernandez Aguilar, G. Choufani, and S. Hassid, "Respiratory epithelial adenomatoid hamartoma associated with nasal polyposis," *Am. J. Otolaryngol*, vol. 25, n° 4, pp. 282-284, July 2004, doi: 10.1016/j.amjoto.2004.02.005.

[183]Z. Cao, Z. Gu, J. Yang, and M. Jin, "Respiratory epithelial adenomatoid hamartoma of bilateral olfactory clefts associated with nasal polyposis: Three cases report and literature review," *Auris. Nasus. Larynx*, vol. 37, nº 3, p. 352-356, June 2010, doi: 10.1016/j.anl.2009.10.003.

[184]E. Masson, "Nasosinus polyposis in adults," *EM-Consulte.* https://www.em-consulte.com/article/19331/polypose-nasosinusienne-chez-l-adulte (accessed June 07, 2019).

[185]M. M. Glovsky, "Upper airways involvement in bronchial asthma," *Curr. Opin. Pulm. Med.* vol. 4, nº 1, pp. 54-58, Jan. 1998.

[186]K. Morwood, D. Gillis, W. Smith, and F. Kette, "Aspirin-sensitive asthma," *Intern. Med. J.*, vol. 35, nº 4, pp. 240-246, Apr. 2005, doi: 10.1111/j.1445-5994.2004.00801.x.

[187]R. G. Slavin, "Nasal polyps and sinusitis," *JAMA*, vol. 278, nº 22, pp. 1849-1854, Dec. 1997.

[188]C. Parietti-Winkler, C. Baumann, P. Gallet, G. Gauchard, and R. Jankowski, "Otitis media with effusion as a marker of the inflammatory process associated to nasal polyposis", *Rhinology*, vol. 47, nº 4, pp. 396-399, Dec. 2009, doi: 10.4193/Rhin08.220.

[189]C. Parietti-Winkler and R. Jankowski, "Is there an association between otitis media and nasal polyposis?", *Curr. Allergy Asthma Rep.* vol. 11, nº 6, pp. 521-525, Dec. 2011, doi: 10.1007/s11882-011-0229-0.

[190]M. Daval *et al*, "Chronic otitis media with effusion in chronic sinusitis with polyps," *Ear. Nose. Throat J.*, vol. 97, nº 8, p. E13-E18, August 2018, doi: 10.1177/014556131809700803.

[191]B. F. Marple, "Allergic fungal rhinosinusitis: current theories and management strategies", *The Laryngoscope*, vol. 111, nº 6, pp. 1006-1019, June 2001, doi: 10.1097/00005537-200106000-00015.

[192]J. Percodani *et al*, "Does allergic fungal sinusitis exist? Preliminary results of a prospective study," *Ann. Oto-Laryngol. Chir. Cervico Faciale Bull. Soc. Oto-Laryngol. Hopitaux Paris*, vol. 116, nº 2, p. 78-84, May 1999.

[193]B. Nussenbaum, B. F. Marple, and N. D. Schwade, "Characteristics of bony erosion in allergic fungal rhinosinusitis," *Otolaryngol.--Head Neck Surg. Off. J. Am. Acad. Otolaryngol.-Head Neck Surg.* vol. 124, nº 2, p. 150-154, Feb. 2001, doi: 10.1067/mhn.2001.112573.

[194]H. Stammberger, R. Jakse, and F. Beaufort, "Aspergillosis of the paranasal sinuses x-ray diagnosis, histopathology, and clinical aspects," *Ann. Otol. Rhinol. Laryngol.* vol. 93, nº 3 Pt 1, pp. 251-256, June 1984, doi: 10.1177/000348948409300313.

[195]S. C. Manning, M. Merkel, K. Kriesel, F. Vuitch, and B. Marple, "Computed tomography and magnetic resonance diagnosis of

allergic fungal sinusitis," *The Laryngoscope*, vol. 107, nº 2, pp. 170-176, Feb. 1997.

[196]M. Mossa-Basha, A. T. Ilica, F. Maluf, Ö. Karakoç, I. Izbudak, and N. Aygün, "The many faces of fungal disease of the paranasal sinuses: CT and MRI findings", *Diagn. Interv. Radiol. Ank. Turk.* vol. 19, nº 3, pp. 195-200, June 2013, doi: 10.5152/dir.2012.003.

[197]S. C. Manning, S. D. Schaefer, L. G. Close, and F. Vuitch, "Culture-positive allergic fungal sinusitis," *Arch. Otolaryngol. Head Neck Surg.* vol. 117, nº 2, pp. 174-178, Feb. 1991.

[198]R. C. Michael, J. S. Michael, R. H. Ashbee, and M. S. Mathews, "Mycological profile of fungal sinusitis: An audit of specimens over a 7-year period in a tertiary care hospital in Tamil Nadu", *Indian J. Pathol. Microbiol*, vol. 51, nº 4, p. 493-496, Dec. 2008.

[199]" Comprehensive management of allergic fungal sinusitis. - PubMed - NCBI." https://www.ncbi.nlm.nih.gov/pubmed/9740919 (accessed June 26, 2019).

[200]" Cystic fibrosis mortality and survival in the UK: 1947-2003. - PubMed - NCBI." https://www.ncbi.nlm.nih.gov/pubmed/17182652 (accessed June 29, 2019).

[201]" Nasal and Sinus Polyposis in Children - Triglia - 1997 - The Laryngoscope - Wiley Online Library." https://onlinelibrary.wiley.com/doi/abs/10.1097/00005537-199707000-00025 (accessed June 29, 2019).

[202]" Nasal polypectomy and sinus surgery for cystic fibrosis--a 10 year review. - PubMed - NCBI." https://www.ncbi.nlm.nih.gov/pubmed/?term=affe+BF%2C+Strome+M%2C+Khaw+KT%2C+Shwachman+H.+Nasal+polypectomy+and+sinus+surgery+for+cystic+fibrosis-a-10+year+review.+Otolaryngol+Clin+North+Am+1977+%3B+10+%3A+81-90 (accessed June 30, 2019).

[203]" Endoscopic sinus surgery in the treatment of cystic fibrosis with nasal polyposis. - PubMed - NCBI." https://www.ncbi.nlm.nih.gov/pubmed/8948619 (accessed June 29, 2019).

[204]" Defining and describing airways obstruction in children. - PubMed - NCBI." https://www.ncbi.nlm.nih.gov/pubmed/?term=Kerrebijn+KF.+Defining+and+describing+airways+obstruction+in+children.+Eur+Respir+J+1990+%3B+3+%3A+1083-1084 (accessed June 29, 2019).

[205]M. Rollin, K. Seymour, M. Hariri, and J. Harcourt, "Rhinosinusitis, symptomatology & absence of polyposis in children with primary ciliary dyskinesia," *Rhinology*, vol. 47, nº 1, pp. 75-78, March 2009.

[206]J. J. Braun, L. Donato, A. Clavert, C. Cranz, L. Hoffmann, and A. Gentine, "Primary ciliary dyskinesia: Clinical study and diagnosis,"

Ann. Otolaryngol. Chir. Cervico-Faciale, vol. 122, n° 2, pp. 63-68, Apr. 2005, doi: 10.1016/S0003-438X(05)82326-6.

[207] C. Werner *et al*, "An international registry for primary ciliary dyskinesia," *Eur. Respir. J.*, vol. 47, n° 3, pp. 849-859, March 2016, doi: 10.1183/13993003.00776-2015.

[208] Woakes E., "Necrotizing ethmoiditis and mucous polyps", *Lancet*, n° 61, 1885.

[209] Canuyt M, Terracol J., " La polypose nasal récidivante et déformante des jeunes ", *Rev Laryng Otol*, n° 45, p. 7-10., 1924.

[210] Busca GP., "The Woakes' syndrome: Ethiopathogenetic and clinical considerations with personal case report", *Minerva Otorinolaringol*, n° 16, p. 201-5, 1966.

[211] U. Schoenenberger and A.-J. Tasman, "Adult-Onset Woakes' Syndrome: Report of a Rare Case," *Case Rep. Otolaryngol.* vol. 2015, pp. 1-4, Apr. 2015, doi: 10.1155/2015/857675.

[212] " Woakes' syndrome and albinism - PDF Free Download," *kundoc.com.* https://kundoc.com/pdf-woakes-syndrome-and-albinism-.html (accessed July 01, 2019).

[213] B. Kellerhals and B. de Uthemann, "Woakes' syndrome: The problems of infantile nasal polyps," *Int. J. Pediatr. Otorhinolaryngol.* vol. 1, n° 1, pp. 79-85, July 1979, doi: 10.1016/0165-5876(79)90031-4.

[214] R. Pialoux, L. Coffinet, J. Derelle, and R. Jankowski, "La polypose naso-sinusienne idiopathique de l'enfant existe-t-elle?", *Arch. Pediatrics*, vol. 6, n° 4, pp. 391-397, Apr. 1999, doi: 10.1016/S0929-693X(99)80220-6.

[215] N. Leboulanger, "Nasal obstruction in children," *Eur. Ann. Otorhinolaryngol. Head Neck Dis.*, vol. 133, n° 3, pp. 183-186, June 2016, doi: 10.1016/j.anorl.2015.09.011.

[216] Triglia J, Bellus J., "La polypose naso-sinusienne de l'enfant: diagnostic et pro-blèmes thérapeutiques", *Ann Pediatr*, n° 39, p. 473-7, 1992.

[217] G. Kanny *et al*, "La rhinite non allergique à éosinophiles ou NARES Aspects cliniques et immunohistologiques", *Rev. Fr. D39Allergologie D39Immunologie Clin*, vol. 38, n° 7, p. 624-633.

[218] D. A. Moneret-Vautrin, R. Jankowski, and M. Wayoff, "[Clinical and pathogenic aspects of NARES (non-allergic rhinitis with eosinophilic syndrome)]", *Rev. Laryngol. - Otol. - Rhinol.* vol. 112, n° 1, pp. 41-44, 1991.

[219] R. Collado-Chagoya *et al*, "[Non-allergic rhinitis with eosinophilic syndrome. Case report]", *Rev. Alerg. Mex. Tecamachalco Puebla Mex. 1993*, vol. 65, n° 3, pp. 310-315, Sept. 2018, doi: 10.29262/ram.v65i3.336.

[220] Moneret-Vautrin D, Jankowski R, Bene M, et al, "NARES: a model of inflammationcaused by activated eosinophils?", *Rhinology*, n° 30, pp. 161-8, 1992.

Chapitre 10 : Differential diagnosis

In its advanced, bilateral form, the differential diagnosis of PNS does not arise. Clinical signs, endoscopic examination and CT scan are sufficient to make the diagnosis of polyposis; in its unilateral or asymmetric form, other diagnoses must be ruled out. [140]

10.1 Bilateral chronic oedematopurulent sinusitis:

The distinction between bilateral nasal polyposis and oedematopurulent sinusitis requires the presence of the following arguments [131] :

- edematous lesions mainly in the middle meatus, and exceptionally in the olfactory slits; they are mixed with purulent secretions in the middle meatus, or give the appearance of dirty secretions disseminated in the nasal cavities;

- directed antibiotic treatment does not prevent the rapid reproduction and clogging of the nasal cavities by pathological secretions, whereas it is capable of cleaning out superinfected polyposis and restoring its typical endoscopic presentation;

- CT scans always reveal frank opacities of the maxillary or frontal sinuses, associated with ethmoidal opacities sometimes limited to the anterior ethmoid.

The clinical picture can be refined by looking for dental infections, immune deficiency, bronchiectasis or chronic bronchitis.

10.2 Churg-Strauss disease:

Also known as eosinophilic granulomatosis with polyangiitis (EGPA), this is a necrotizing systemic vasculitis of small and medium-sized vessels, characterized by asthma and blood eosinophilia. It may present as an infected polyposis or bilateral oedematopurulent sinusitis, but is usually associated with asthma, altered general condition, febrile syndrome or other localizations (lung, heart, prostate, skin...). [221,222]

10.3 Bilateral antrochoanal polyp:

The typical unilateral antrochoanal polyp with an antral (maxillary) cystic component and a nasal or choanal fleshy polyp is the most frequent presentation of sinuso-choanal polyps (antro-, sphenoido-, or fronto-choanal).

Confusion may arise with nasal polyposis when they develop bilaterally, or when contralateral ethmoidal opacities are associated with a unilateral form, in which case surgical intervention can usually rectify the diagnosis by emptying contralateral ethmoidal retention secretions. Bilateral presentation is extremely rare, with only a handful of cases reported in the literature. [154,223,224]

10.4 Chronic respiratory rhinitis:

In forms of allergic rhinitis evolving for several years without treatment, nasal endoscopy reveals mucous hypersecretion, with major hypertrophy of the lower turbinates associated with edema of the free edge of the middle turbinates, suggesting nasal polyposis. A CT scan rectifies the diagnosis, showing in allergic rhinitis an ethmoid and paranasal sinuses without pathological opacity, while the two respiratory passages appear considerably narrowed, sometimes virtual. [225,131]

10.5 Inverted papilloma:

Inverted papilloma is a benign epithelial tumor of slow and rare evolution, preferentially affecting adults in the fifth decade. [226]

Its etiology remains poorly understood to this day, but it has been reported to be associated with human papillomavirus in almost 40% of cases, raising suspicion of its role in the pathogenesis of inverted papilloma. Treatment is by endoscopic endonasal or external surgery. [227,228]

The initial location is highly characteristic: lateral wall of the nasal cavity, turbinates and middle meatus, sometimes nasal septum. This is a unilateral nasoethmoido-maxillary mass, with localized bone destruction.

Clinical and radiological doubt leads to biopsy with anatomopathological examination of all excised material. [15]

10.6 Epitheliomas of the ethmoid :

Most often of occupational origin in woodworkers. Initially unilateral or predominantly unilateral. It then spreads to the orbit and the anterior part of the skull base. [11]

Clinically, the combination of a history of occupational exposure and epistaxis suggests the need for a biopsy.

Radiologically, the lesions are localized in a single ethmoido-nasal sector on CT. MRI is invaluable in differentiating between inflammatory and neoplastic processes. [15]

10.7 Angiomatous polyps and nasopharyngeal fibroma :

Angiomatous polyps are simply thickenings of the mucous membrane of the nasal cavity, but their vascularization can be quite extensive, giving them a hemorrhagic character.

On CT scan, after injection of contrast medium, the enhancement is of low density, as in Killian's polyp, and therefore has nothing in common with the massive contrast enhancement seen in nasopharyngeal fibroids, which are also centred on the spheno-palatine foramen. It occurs in adolescent males, and the frequency and abundance of epistaxis point to this diagnosis. Surgical management usually requires embolization in the 72 hours prior to surgery.

10.8 Esthesioneuroblastomas:

It is a rare malignant tumor, developing from the neurosensory cells of the olfactory mucosa. Ocular involvement, which is often rhinological, may be inaugural or occur during the evolution of secondary orbital involvement. [229,230]

The lesion is heterogeneous, contrast-enhancing on CT, and may present with calcifications and lysis of the ethmoid sieve blade. Diagnosis is anatomopathological, and treatment usually involves surgery followed by radiotherapy. [231,232]

References :

[11] Mahassine EL HARRAS, "la polypose nasosinusienne: place de la chirurgie endonasale", Université CADI AYYAD, Marrakech, 2011.

[15] SOULTANA RABIE, "nasosinusal polyposis: experience of the ENT department at Moulay Ismail Hospital in Meknes (à propos de 60 cas)", Université Sidi Mohammed ben Abdellah, FES, 2015.

[131] R. Jankowski, C. Rumeau, P. Gallet, and D. T. Nguyen, "Nasal polyposis (or chronic olfactory rhinitis)," *Ann. Fr. Oto-Rhino-Laryngol. Pathol. Cervico-Faciale*, vol. 135, n° 3, pp. 190-196, June 2018, doi: 10.1016/j.aforl.2017.09.014.

[140] P. Dessi and F. Facon, "Nasosinus polyposis in adults", *Encycl Méd Chir Oto-rhino-laryngologie*, p. 16, 2003.

[154] Y. F. Yilmaz, A. Titiz, M. Ozcan, M. S. Tezer, S. Ozlugedik, and A. Unal, "Bilateral antrochoanal polyps in an adult: a case report", *B-ENT*, vol. 3, n° 2, pp. 97-99, 2007.

[221] A. T. Masi *et al*, "The American College of Rheumatology 1990 criteria for the classification of Churg-Strauss syndrome (allergic granulomatosis and angiitis)", *Arthritis Rheum.* vol. 33, n° 8, pp. 1094-1100, August 1990.

[222] Y. Nguyen and L. Guillevin, "Eosinophilic Granulomatosis with Polyangiitis (Churg-Strauss)," *Semin. Respir. Crit. Care Med.* vol. 39, n° 4, pp. 471-481, 2018, doi: 10.1055/s-0038-1669454.

[223] P. Singhal and N. Gupta, "Bilateral Antrochoanal Polyp in an Adult: A Rarity," *Clin. Rhinol. Int. J.*, vol. 4, pp. 145-146, Sept. 2011, doi: 10.5005/jp-journals-10013-1095.

[224] O. Iziki, S. Rouadi, R. L. Abada, M. Roubal, and M. Mahtar, "Bilateral antrochoanal polyp: report of a new case and systematic review of the literature," *J. Surg. Case Rep.* vol. 2019, n° 3, p. rjz074, March 2019, doi: 10.1093/jscr/rjz074.

[225] R. Jankowski, D. T. Nguyen, A. Russel, B. Toussaint, P. Gallet, and C. Rumeau, "Chronic nasal dysfunction," *Ann. Fr. Oto-Rhino-Laryngol. Pathol. Cervico-Faciale*, vol. 135, n° 1, pp. 43-51, Feb. 2018, doi: 10.1016/j.aforl.2017.08.008.

[226] M. Chihani, K. Nadour, M. Touati, Y. Darouassi, H. Ammar, and B. Bouaity, "Inverted papilloma: retrospective study about 22 cases", *Pan Afr. Med. J.*, vol. 17, March 2014, doi: 10.11604/pamj.2014.17.208.3936.

[227] Q. Lisan, O. Laccourreye, and P. Bonfils, "Inverted nasosinusal papilloma: from diagnosis to treatment," *Ann. Fr. Oto-Rhino-Laryngol. Pathol. Cervico-Faciale*, vol. 133, n° 5, pp. 304-309, Nov. 2016, doi: 10.1016/j.aforl.2015.12.004.

[228] M. Ben Amor *et al*, "Nasosinus inverted papilloma: 43 cases", *Presse Médicale*, vol. 42, n° 6, Part 1, pp. e171-e176, June 2013, doi: 10.1016/j.lpm.2012.11.008.
[229] A. Lapierre, I. Selmaji, H. Samlali, T. Brahmi, and S. Yossi, "Esthesioneuroblastoma: retrospective study and review of the literature", *Cancer/Radiotherapy*, vol. 20, n° 8, pp. 783-789, Dec. 2016, doi: 10.1016/j.canrad.2016.05.015.
[230] G. Klironomos *et al*, "Endoscopic management of Esthesioneuroblastoma: Our experience and review of the literature", *J. Clin. Neurosci.* vol. 58, pp. 117-123, Dec. 2018, doi: 10.1016/j.jocn.2018.09.011.
[231] M. Kriet *et al*, "Esthesioneuroblastoma olfactory of ophthalmologic revelation," */data/revues/01815512/00250006/632/*, March 2008, Accessed: Jul 12, 2019. [Online]. Available from: https://www.em-consulte.com/en/article/112429.
[232] B. Fiani *et al*, "Esthesioneuroblastoma: A Comprehensive Review of Diagnosis, Management, and Current Treatment Options," *World Neurosurg.* vol. 126, pp. 194-211, June 2019, doi: 10.1016/j.wneu.2019.03.014.

Chapitre 11 : Evolution

11.1 Untreated:

If left untreated, the nasal polyps would continue to evolve and grow in volume, until externalization through the nostrils at the front or through the choanae into the cavum at the back.

Deformity of the nasal canopy may be observed, with aesthetic damage and the possibility of locoregional complications, in particular orbital complications such as exophthalmos, dacryocystitis and even spontaneous mucoceles due to blocked drainage of the sinus cavities, favored by frequent superinfections.

Symptomatology, particularly nasosinus symptoms, worsens. Nasal obstruction and anosmia become bothersome, with an impact on quality of life that deteriorates further and further, leading to a negative effect on the patient's socio-professional life.

11.2 Under treatment :

With proper medical or surgical treatment and patient compliance, polyp pathology can be stabilized and patients' quality of life improved, particularly after surgery. This is reflected in quality-of-life scores on quality-of-life evaluation tests, which are lower than pre-treatment scores, as assessed by several publications.

Despite well-administered medical and surgical treatment, recurrences are sometimes inevitable and frequent, necessitating repeated interventions.

11.2.1 Overall symptomatic efficacy:

Overall analysis of the efficacy of medical-surgical treatment in series analyzing only patients with PNS, shows improvement in 37% to 99% of cases, with an average of 89%. Analysis of the results shows that the longer the follow-up, the worse the results. [29]

11.2.2 Effective on all symptoms:

11.2.2.1 Anosmia:

Smell disorders are not always clearly improved after surgical treatment, with some authors reporting better improvement in the sense of smell with radical surgery than with functional surgery. Overall, however, good surgical results on the sense of smell deteriorate with time. [233]

All studies report an improvement in postoperative sense of smell ranging from 13 to 91%, with a median of 31%. [234]

11.2.2.2 Nasal obstruction

The effectiveness of endonasal surgery in improving nasal obstruction has been proven by several studies, with this symptom being most consistently and durably improved by surgical treatment.

All series show improvement from 29 to 100% with a mean of 72%. [234]

11.2.2.3 Rhinorrhea :

This symptom is most often improved by surgical treatment.

11.2.2.4 Facial pain :

They may exist before any surgical procedure, or appear postoperatively, but their evolution is usually favorable over time.

11.2.2.5 Progression of asthma :

Several authors confirm the stabilization of asthma after treatment of SFN, either through a reduction in attacks, or a reduction in therapeutic doses and the use of corticosteroid treatments. [235,236]

11.2.2.6 Quality of life :

Several authors have shown an improvement in the quality of life of patients with nasosinusal polyposis, both after medical treatment and after surgical cure. [237,238]

11.2.2.7 Recidivism :

Post-operative recurrences of nasosinusal polyposis are frequent.

The literature review found variable recurrence rates, this variability may be due to the length of follow-up, in the literature the recurrence rate varies from 8% to 66% with a median of 25% for Bonfils [140] Elkorbi 23% [239] Rombaux 40% [240].

The variability in endoscopic recurrence rates can be explained by the nature of post-operative management and the quality of patient compliance.

Their occurrence varies:

- Early recurrences, less than a year old, are observed in patients with fragile conditions such as asthma or Widal's disease. Their treatment often involves medical therapies, sometimes combined with local procedures such as polypectomy under local anaesthetic.

- Late recurrences: These are increasingly common, and are treated by repeat surgery under general anaesthetic.

References :

[29] R. Jankowski, *Du dysfonctionnement naso-sinusien chronique au dysfonctionnement ostio-meatal*. Paris: Société Française d'Oto-rhino-laryngologie et de Chrurgie de la Face et du Cou, 2006.

[140] P. Dessi and F. Facon, "Nasosinus polyposis in adults", *Encycl Méd Chir Oto-rhino-laryngologie*, p. 16, 2003.

[233] R. Jankowski, D. Pigret, and F. Decroocq, "Comparison of functional results after ethmoidectomy and nasalization for diffuse and severe nasal polyposis," *Acta Otolaryngol. (Stockh.)*, vol. 117, n° 4, p. 601-608, July 1997, doi: 10.3109/00016489709113445.

[234] K. Dalziel, K. Stein, A. Round, R. Garside, and P. Royle, "Systematic review of endoscopic sinus surgery for nasal polyps," *Health Technol. Assess. Winch. Engl.* vol. 7, n° 17, p. iii, 1-159, 2003.

[235] " Effects of Sinus Surgery on Asthma in Aspirin Triad Patients: Acta Oto-Laryngologica: Vol 119, No 5."

https://www.tandfonline.com/doi/abs/10.1080/00016489950180856?journalCode=ioto20 (accessed Sept. 23, 2019).
[236] T. A. Loehrl, R. M. Ferre, R. J. Toohill, and T. L. Smith, "Long-term asthma outcomes after endoscopic sinus surgery in aspirin triad patients," *Am. J. Otolaryngol.* vol. 27, n° 3, pp. 154-160, June 2006, doi: 10.1016/j.amjoto.2005.09.001.
[237] F. Radenne *et al*, "Quality of life in nasal polyposis☆☆☆★," *J. Allergy Clin. Immunol.* vol. 104, n° 1, pp. 79-84, July 1999, doi: 10.1016/S0091-6749(99)70117-X.
[238] " [Quality of life before and after surgery in patients with nasal polyposis]. - ClinicalKey.html".
[239] A. El korbi, N. Kolsi, B. Alaya, Z. Ben rhaiem, K. Harrathi, and J. Koubaa, "Nasosinusal polyposis: are there predictive factors for recurrence after surgical treatment?", *121st Congress 2014 October 11-13 Paris - Palais Congrès*, vol. 131, n° 4, Supplement, p. A155, Oct. 2014, doi: 10.1016/j.aforl.2014.07.359.
[240] P. Rombaux, C. de Toeuf, M. Hamoir, P. Eloy, and B. Bertrand, "La polypose naso-sinusienne," *Ann Otolaryngol Chir Cervicofac*, vol. 118, p. 8, 2001.

Conclusion:

Nasosinusal polyposis is a complex, disabling inflammatory disease of the nasosinus cavities, characterized by a tendency to recur despite well-managed medical and surgical treatment. This multifactorial pathology, the cause of which is still poorly understood, is a benign condition that does not degenerate, but is progressive and recurrent.

Nasosinus polyposis predominates in young adults, and is part of a group of chronic inflammatory diseases of the respiratory mucosa. As a result, asthma, aspirin intolerance and respiratory allergy should be systematically investigated. The rarer paediatric forms of the condition should be investigated for mucociliary dysfunction or cystic fibrosis. Diagnosis of this condition has greatly benefited from the advent and progress of endoscopy and CT imaging. Management is always medical, sometimes surgical, depending on the patient's functional discomfort and quality of life, the clinical and paraclinical presentation of the pathology itself, co-morbidity and, above all, the socio-professional impact and wishes of the patient.

List of abbreviations

5-HPETE : Acide 5-HydroPeroxyEicosaTetraEnoïque.

ADN : Acide DésoxyriboNucléique

AINS : Anti-Inflammatoires Non Stéroïdiens.

CO2 : Dioxyde de carbone.

COX : Cyclo-oxygénase.

CRS : Chronic Rhino-Sinusitis : rhinosinusite chronique.

CSF : Colony Stimulating Factor.

EFR : Exploration Fonctionnelle Respiratoire.

EGPA : Eosinophilic Granulomatosis with PolyAngiitis.

EMCRS : Eosinophil Mycotic Chronic Rhino-Sinusitis.

EO : Eotaxin.

ESA : Entérotoxines de Staphylococcus Aureus.

EVA : Echelle Visuelle Analogique.

FDA : Food and Drug Administration.

FESS : Functional Endoscopic Sinus Surgery.

GM-CSF : Granulocyte-Macrophage Colony-Stimulating Factor.

HERA : Hamartomes Epithéliaux Respiratoires Adénomatoïdes.

HLA-DR : Complexe majeur d'histocompatibilité de type II.

ICAM-1 : Inter-Cellular Adhesion Molecule-1.

IFN : Interféron.

IL : Interleukine.

IRM : Imagerie par Résonance Magnétique.

KTP : Potassium-Titanyl-Phosphate.

LCR : Liquide Céphalo-Rachidien.

LCS : Liquide Cérébro-Spinal.

LT : Leucotriène.

MRV : Mixed Respiratory Vaccine.

NALT : Nasal Associated Lymphoid Tissue.

NAORES : Non-Allergic Olfactory Rhinitis with Eosinophilia Syndrome.

NARES : Non Allergic Rhinitis Eosinophil Syndrome.

NO : Oxyde Nitrique.

O2 : Oxygène.

OMS : Organisation Mondiale de la Santé.

PNN : Poly-Nucléaires Neutrophiles.

PNS : Polypose Naso-Sinusienne.

QdV : Qualité de Vie.

QoL : Quality of Life.

RANTES : Regulated on Activation Normal T cells Expressed and Secreted.

RhinoQoL : Rhinosinusitis Quality of Life Survey.

RSFA : Rhino>-Sinusite Fongique Allergique.

SCF : Stem Cell Factor.

SNOT-16-ARS : Sino-Nasal Outcome Test-16 modifié pour la rhinosinusite aigue.

SNOT-20 : Sino-Nasal Outcome Test-20.

SNOT-22 : Sino-Nasal Outcome Test-22.

Std Dev : Deviation standard.

TDM : Tomo-Densito-Métrie.

TGF : Transforming Growth Factor.

TGF-b1 : Transforming Growth Factor beta 1.

TH : T Helper.

TNF-a : Tumor Necrosis Factor alpha.

TSLP : Stroma thymique dérivé de cellules épithéliales lymphopoïétine.

UCTMR : Unité de Contrôle de la Tuberculose et des Maladies Respiratoires.

USA : United States of América.

VEMS : Volume Expiratoire Maximal par Seconde.

YAG : Ytrium-Aluminium-Garnet.

Table of contents

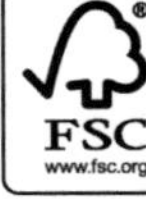

MIX
Papier aus verantwortungsvollen Quellen
Paper from responsible sources
FSC® C105338

Printed by Books on Demand GmbH, Norderstedt / Germany